Healthcare Information Systems: Challenges of the New Millennium

Adi Armoni
Tel Aviv College of Management, Israel

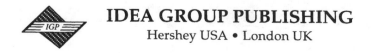
IDEA GROUP PUBLISHING
Hershey USA • London UK

Senior Editor: Mehdi Khosrowpour
Managing Editor: Jan Travers
Copy Editor: Maria M. Boyer
Typesetter: Tamara Gillis
Cover Design: Connie Peltz
Printed at: BookCrafters

Published in the United States of America by
        Idea Group Publishing
        1331 E. Chocolate Avenue
        Hershey PA 17033-1117
        Tel: 717-533-8845
        Fax: 717-533-8661
        E-mail: jtravers@idea-group.com
        Website: http://www.idea-group.com

and in the United Kingdom by
        Idea Group Publishing
        3 Henrietta Street
        Covent Garden
        London WC2E 8LU
        Tel: 171-240 0856
        Fax: 171-379 0609
        http://www.eurospan.co.uk

Library of Congress Cataloging-in-Publication Data

Armoni, Adi, 1959-
    Healthcare information systems : challenges of the new millennium / Adi Armoni.
        p. cm.
    Includes bibliographical references and index
    ISBN 1-878289-62-4 (pbk.)
        1. Information storage and retrieval systems --Medical care. 2. Medical
    informatics. I. Title.
    R858 .A76 2000
    362.1'0285--dc21   99-052784

British Cataloguing in Publication Data
A Cataloguing in Publication record for this book is available from the British Library.

NEW from Idea Group Publishing

Healthcare Information Systems: Challenges of the New Millennium

Table of Contents

Preface

Information technology application in healthcare has a long history, triggered from two separate areas of interest. On the one hand, the development of medical instruments has incorporated information technology in a vast number of instances, varying from monitor equipment to CT and MRI scanners. On the other hand, requirements on the registration and processing of medical services and hospital bills, often imposed by government or insurance companies, have led to extensive Electronic Data Processing facilities (EDP), Hospital Information Systems (HIS) and ancillary registration systems.

These two areas of information technology applications in healthcare, are rapidly integrating, starting with local integration between, for example, Laboratory Information Management Systems, which interface and integrate different kinds of analyzers, and laboratory registration systems which keep track of patients, orders, results, and bills. Increasingly, clinical workstations are being developed which interface with variety of systems (HIS, Lab, Radiology, Medical Records, ATD, etc.), and should be accessible to number of different users (physicians, nurses, etc.).

This wide variety of platforms, data needs to support the medical decision-making processes, ethical and legal aspects, various kinds of application and users, poses an enormous challenge to the field of healthcare information technology and promises to keep it at the edge of the information innovation revolution.

Given the tremendous increase in the amount of data and computerization of information resources, competence is no longer characterized by the amount of knowledge held in the memory of the clinician, but as the ability to properly utilize databases and other on-line electronic data sources. The book consists of 10 excellent chapters covering the main issues leading the innovation revolution in information technology in medicine. Among those issues the reader may find a wide coverage of the following fields:

Information Security

This chapter outlines the major issues related to the security of the medical information systems. Medical information systems are unique in this sense that integrity of the records and privacy issues are dominant. The presentation includes the formulation of the basic medical information security tenets as well as the discussion of the major components of the security subsytem: patient identification, access mechanism, reference monitor, communication subsystem and database subsystem. Also examples of privacy law are quoted and discussed.

Success and Failure of Healthcare Information Systems

Some healthcare information systems do succeed, but the majority are likely to fail in some way. New information systems have a powerful potential to improve the functioning of healthcare organizations. However, that potential can only be realized if healthcare information systems can be successfully developed and implemented. To explain why this happens and how failure rates may be reduced, the chapter describes a model of conception—reality gaps. This argues that the greater the change gap between current realities and the design conceptions (i.e. requirements and assumptions) of a new healthcare information system, the greater the risk of failure.

Three archetypal large design-reality gaps affect the healthcare information systems domain and are associated with an increased risk of failure:

- Rationality-reality gaps: that arise from the formal, rational way in which many healthcare information systems are conceived, which mismatches the behavioral realities of some healthcare organizations.
- Private-public sector gaps: that arise from application in public sector contexts of healthcare information systems developed for the private sector.
- Country gaps: that arise from application in one country of healthcare information systems developed in a different country.

Some generic conclusions can be drawn about successful approaches to healthcare information systems development.

Telemedicine

Health systems take on new meaning in the midst of the international communication revolution going on. Health services are a natural candidate to join and even become an integral part of the "Information Highway." Terms such as telemedicine, telehealth, teleradiology, teledermatology, etc., have been integrated into technical and academic jargon and have become the object of research and organization.

The two central components effect the success of telemedicine assimilation are the cost of the service and the quality of service. Acceptance of telemedicine in the life of the individual and the organisation will demand a substantial change in clinical and organisational conceptions, and will result in a revolution in the existing accepted health organisation structure, in treatment and diagnosis procedures, and in the health system policy as a whole.

Methods for Handling Complexity in Hospital Information Systems

Anyone working in the area of hospital information systems is sooner or later amazed about the intrinsic complexity of the field. Finding ways to handle this complexity seems utterly important. In this chapter the author presents a user-oriented, document-based approach being developed and proven in cooperation projects with hospitals. The advantage of the proposed approach lies in the provision of means for handling different sources of complexity. The approach is characterized by an intended continuous switch between an organizational and workplace perspective in order to reduce complexity by changing the levels of detail.

Artificial Intelligence in Medicine

In recent years we have witnessed sweeping developments in information technology. Currently, the most promising and interesting domain seemed to be the artificial intelligence. Within this field we see now a growing interest in the medical applications. The purpose of this article is to present a general review of the main areas of artificial intelligence and its applications to the medical domain. The review will focus on artificial intelligence applications to radiology, robotically-operated surgical procedures and different kinds of expert systems.

Knowledge acquisition and the evaluation of retrieved probabilities
The chapter examines the behavior of the human decision-maker. It surveys research in which about 90 physicians specializing in various fields and with different degrees of seniority participated. It tackles the question of whether it is possible to found the majority of the knowledge bases of the expert systems on the Bayesian theory. We will discuss the way of decision making conforming to the probabilities evaluated according to the Bayesian theory.

I am sure that this book offers a significant contribution to the physicians, information systems experts and for all personnel that uses healthcare information technology.

Acknowledgments

Putting together a book of this level requires a tremendous effort and hard work. I greatly appreciate the valuable help from the authors and my reviewers for their excellent contributions to this book. I also greatly appreciate the assistance of managing editor, Ms. Jan Travers at Idea Group Publishing. And of course, without the strong support of my family Ronit, Ran, Guy, and Tamar Armoni, this book would never be possible.

Adi Armoni
September 1999

Chapter I

Designing Hospital Information Systems: Handling Complexity via a User-Oriented Document-Based Approach

Anita Krabbel and Ingrid Wetzel
University of Hamburg, Germany

Anyone working in the area of hospital information systems is sooner or later amazed about the intrinsic complexity of the field. Finding ways to handle this complexity seems utterly important. In this chapter we present a user-oriented, document-based approach being developed and proven in cooperation projects with hospitals. The advantage of the proposed approach lies in the provision of means for handling different sources of complexity. The approach is characterized by an intended continuous switch between an organizational and workplace perspective in order to reduce complexity by changing the levels of detail. It initiates and supports ongoing negotiation processes among the heterogeneous user groups by providing user-oriented, easy-to-understand documents. Furthermore, it enables developers and users alike to represent and discuss current and future work practices including interim solutions of future system support.

INTRODUCTION

Those working in the domain of hospital information systems (HIS) are quite soon amazed or upset about the intrinsic complexity of the field. To change only a small part in the organization of a task often requires an overwhelming amount of details to be taken into account. Trying to isolate a section for starting system design seems hopeless because of the interdependence of tasks. Trying to reach agreement on priorities within cross-departmental solutions is tiring due to the heterogeneity of the involved user groups.

Finding ways to handle this complexity is utterly important. A major reason for this complexity lies in the amount of complex cooperations necessary to care for a patient (see also Schneider and Wagner, 1993). This patient is a very sophisticated (and precious), shared material" (but still remaining real and not vanishing in transformation to an electronic model). A patient requires *different specialists* and therefore their coordination, his changing condition demands *flexibility*, sometimes discarding all planned actions. The *location* of a patient changes for shorter or longer periods, but staff still need the ability to locate their patient. A patient needs care on different levels (medical, nursing, hospitality) *around the clock* therefore requiring work shifts with their own communication needs. And above all, there is not only one patient but many of them.

Out of those concerns we identify three important aspects which need to be considered and handled by an appropriate approach for analysis and design of HIS.

- First, because of the high amount of existing cooperative work, designers need to understand the relationships and interdependencies among single activities. They have to identify and understand joint, cross-departmental tasks from an organizational perspective and in a broad manner. At the same time, details of work organization and workload within a specific context have to be gathered carefully at each workplace and especially at group workplaces. Additionally, the different perspectives need to be switched frequently (see also Wolf and Karat, 1997). This gives rise to the following guideline: *Handle complexity of cooperative tasks by changing focus and (thereby) levels of abstraction.*
- Second, another source of complexity lies in the heterogeneity of the involved user groups and their often competing requirements, while at the same time designing an integrated system to connect the different groups. Therefore, designers have to take competing wishes into account and be aware of the often hidden power structures in the organization. They have to fight against

narrowed perspectives and, at the same time, endlessly attempting to motivate an integrated solution against possible disadvantages for the individual units. Designers must work out agreeable solutions together with representatives of the different units. This builds another guideline: *Handle complexity of competing requirements by initiating ongoing negotiation processes.*

- A third reason for complexity is closely related to the other two. Implementing an HIS certainly causes changes in the entire work organization. Since hospitals often have little professional focus on organizational development, designers have to initiate (a nonexisting) infrastructure for organizational development together with appropriate techniques. These techniques should provide clear and comprehensive representations of the existing as well as of future work organization along with step-by-step system introduction (see also Wolf and Karat, 1997). This aspect leads to the following guideline: *Handle complexity by providing techniques for illustrating the current and future work practice.*

As pointed out above, an adequate approach for designing HIS must consider these three aspects of complexity. It has to indicate a way to proceed with identification of certain necessary steps or tasks, and provide techniques according to the given guidelines.

The presented approach was worked out in different projects with hospitals. Our main project was devoted to support the decision-finding process of a hospital regarding the development and/or selection respectively of an integrated hospital information system (HIS) in the clinical sections and planning the configuration, introduction, and use of this HIS in the light of changing demands. The cooperation partner was a small acute care hospital with 230 beds and 560 employees. The assignment of the project was embedded in the organizational development in the hospital which has taken place with the participation of all groups of employees from the different departments: internal medicine, surgery, anesthesiology, nursing staff, administration, maintenance/technical support. It started three-and-a-half years ago. We — a team of three computer scientists (one of us being also a nurse) — made a requirements' analysis on the basis of workplace studies and participatory techniques for understanding the cross-departmental processes in the hospital. Out of this and in close cooperation with representatives of the hospital we worked out criteria for the future system and carried out a marked analysis for hospital information systems in Germany. We proposed a system, and after a decision process in the hospital, the system was bought and is now in its customization process. Currently, the system runs in the patient administration, at the wards for the physicians and nurses, and starts to get introduced for communication with the functional working places, like x-ray. Other projects addressed requirements analysis and design for customizable nursing systems and consultant work within a software house building an HIS.

FOUR DIMENSIONS OF OUR USER-ORIENTED, DOCUMENT-BASED APPROACH

Based on our experience in the above mentioned cooperation projects with hospitals, we propose the following approach. It includes four different dimensions, which are briefly introduced at this point and further elucidated throughout the chapter. For the purpose of identification, and combinations of the four dimensions, the following illustrations are presented here. The approach includes:

Dimension 1: An organizational and a workplace perspective.
This dimension follows the first guideline for reducing complexity. As it will be shown, frequent shifts between both perspectives are necessary. Aspects of each perspective can be analyzed in different levels of detail, in selected parts, and with different questions concerning what to consider.

Dimension 2: User-oriented document types.
This dimension corresponds with the second guideline. The user-oriented documents need to be easily understood and useful for

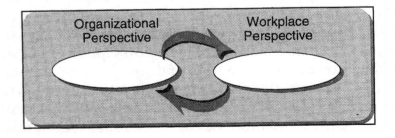

initiating processes among user groups. Nevertheless, each document type must capture a certain aspect concerning analysis and design, and has to support processes for agreement, negotiation (Egger and Wagner, 1993; Simon, Long and Ellis, 1996) and organizational development.

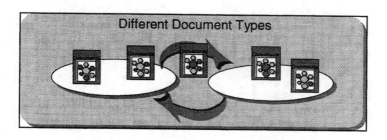

Dimension 3: A focus on current and future work practices.

This dimension is a consequence of the third guideline. In the context of complex cooperation, it is necessary to carefully analyze the current situation. It is important to mirror the current work practices, but even this is quite difficult to achieve. The purpose of cooperation is often a stable element while the "how" of cooperation will change with system support. Therefore, the anticipation of changes during system design is extremely important and demands new techniques (Krabbel, Wetzel Züllighoven, 1997). Prototyping proven useful for single-user systems seems less appropriate for envisioning changes in cooperative settings with all the additional environmental factors. Further more, it is highly valuable to plan and discuss interim solutions necessary due to a stepwise introduction of an integrated system.

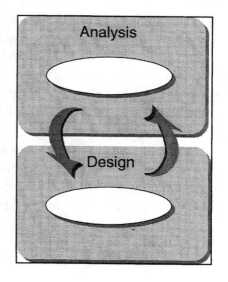

Dimension 4:
An evolutionary way to proceed.

Since complexity reduction can't be accomplished in only one attempt, we certainly need an evolutionary approach. However, each of the steps can

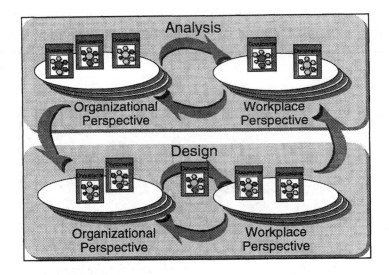

be directed or augmented by clear questions. A new cycle can be devoted to a new investigation or on the basis of reflection and evaluation leading to repeated or deeper analysis.

The approach presented here is founded on the tradition of evolutionary system development, in particular STEPS (Software Technology for Evolutionary Participative Systems development) (Floyd, Reisin and Schmidt, 1989) and the Tools&Materials approach (Bürkle, Gryczan and Züllighoven, 1995; Riehle and Züllighoven, 1995). The emphasis and aims of these approaches lie in evolutionary software development, based on a cyclical process model; in support of a participative communication and learning process for developers and users alike; on the emphasis on the use context, which results in an interlacing of system design and organizational development; on a task-oriented requirements analysis, oriented on the tasks of organizations instead of system functions, as well as in the support perspective, which is expressed in the leitmotif of software workplaces for qualified human activity and views the user as the expert (Floyd, 1987; Floyd, Züllighoven, Budde and Keil-Slawik, 1992). The already proven approaches are by now extended for CSCW, CHI and PDC aspects especially important in the HIS domain.

DOCUMENT TYPES IN DETAIL

The approach is directed by document types which were investigated and used in hospital projects and also in projects from other domains. Each document type is devoted to a certain task and provides a representation of a special aspect in analysis or design. Documents are working material, accompany the entire procedure, and initiate processes which need to take place (Krabbel, Wetzel and Ratuski, 1996). Each document type is easy to understand and can be used by user groups immediately without any agenda or explanation. Their evident simplicity should not conceal the fact that they capture certain aspects in the right abstraction, focus on necessary aspects or bring complex facts to a point.

Our approach for analysis and design is therefore best elucidated by introducing these document types. Each of the document types is described in a uniform way according to the following pattern:

- Contribution to the development process
- Content
- Construction process
- Example
- Project Experience

We structure the presentation by first introducing document types related to analysis and, in a second step describing those needed during design. This is done in spite of the fact that we emphasize a necessary close intertwining of these two activities. Each subsection is further subdivided according to taking up a workplace and an organizational perspective.

Analysis of the Current Work Practice

A good starting point for the analysis of the current work practices is the use of qualitative interviews at workplaces. Interviews are evaluated by producing Scenarios and Glossaries. Due to the heterogeneity of the involved user groups, the organizational perspective with joint tasks requires communicative techniques. For that reason, we introduce Cooperation Pictures and Purpose Tables; for discussing differences among similar workplaces, Task Pictures are used.

For planning interviews, a list of interviews has to be worked out. The interview partners should be chosen following the concept of a functional role. A functional role is classified by a collection of tasks for which a person or a group of persons is responsible. The choice of the concrete interviewees (staff) for each planned functional role should be made by hospital representatives. The interviews should be performed in series and held by small developer teams. This has the advantage of making partial results transparent. Furthermore, each series can be devoted to the investigation of certain relationships in the organizational perspective.

With the technique of qualitative interviews, it is possible to get a profound understanding of the tasks and their performance at certain workplaces. The main focus lies on the learning and communication processes and not in the complete registering of each activity. It is very important that the interviews are held at the actual workplaces in order to get an impression of the entire circumstances. It is worth mentioning that the open form of the interview should not focus on the tasks or functions alone, but also on the necessary established or situated kinds of coordination (Suchman, 1995), or on work distribution and organization, especially in teams.

The evaluation of interviews is performed by writing Scenarios and Glossaries.

Document Types Scenario and Glossary
Contribution to the Development Process

Scenarios and Glossaries belong to the workplace perspective. They are used to evaluate interviews and support the learning process among the developers regarding the work situation of single employees. This includes different aspects: the work tasks and work organization, the used materials and the articulation work (Schmidt and Bannon, 1992). Scenarios and Glossaries are used for feedback with users to identify misunderstandings or lacking aspects. Additionally, interim project results become accessible for the interview partner.

Content

A Scenario describes the present way of accomplishing work tasks with means and objects of work, in the professional language of the user. The main terms are additionally described in a Glossary which might also include example documents. If these documents are available in electronic form, e.g. in an intranet, we augment Glossary entries with scanned documents where possible.

Construction process

The elaboration of Scenarios and Glossaries is done stepwise. As a first step, the developer team has to identify and name tasks based on the interview results. Next, the Scenarios and Glossaries are written. Finally, they get feedback from the interview partners and need a revision.

Example

The example shows a part of the Scenario: "Accompanying and Documenting a Ward Round"

... At least one nurse accompanies the physician during the daily ward round. ...

The ward round takes place every morning. Each patient is visited. The nurse is responsible for carrying the patients' record files.

The physician gives orders for examinations, for changing the medicine, the treatment, the therapy and the care and writes them down on the ward round form. ...

After the ward round the nurse transfers the examination orders to order forms, changes in medicine to the chart, ...

Project Experience

As mentioned above, interviews together with Scenarios and Glossaries, supported us (the analyzing team) in quickly gaining a profound understanding of the context and task performance in the workplaces. Since they are written in the language of the users the feedback cycle gave users the understanding that their knowledge is important for the whole process. Analysts received assurance that their perception was quite appropriate. Some of the users even asked for the description of their tasks to present to their relatives. During each of the phases (even later in the introduction process of the system), the design/selection team returned several times to reread these documents to reinforce detailed information.

For an organizational perspective it is important to understand the interdependencies (Malone and Crowston, 1994) and relationships among tasks being performed at different workplaces. Developers must identify and investigate tasks that expand beyond an individual workplace. From the many single interviews, it is possible to gain an increasing understanding of these joint tasks in the hospital. This includes the identification of interactions among users, but also of gaps and contradictions in Scenarios from different workplaces, e.g., unclearness why something (for instance a document or a piece of information) was passed on to another person or another department, or what the receiver does with it.

At the same time, it becomes apparent that this requires new techniques in order to give feedback of the analysis from the developers to the respective user groups. For this reason, Cooperation Pictures and Purpose Tables were invented (Krabbel, Ratuski and Wetzel, 1996).

Document Type Cooperation Picture

Contribution to the Development Process

Cooperation Pictures promote the understanding, illustration and feedback of the current work practices of joint tasks. They contribute to an acquisition of joint understanding.

Additionally, they support the transition from analysis of the current situation, to system requirements and design. By indicating cooperation density, they provide a valuable basis for defining the application kernel (as described below).

Furthermore, they can be used to discuss and envision changes in the organization of joint tasks.

Content

The focus lies on the representation of how people work together. For that purpose, the passing-on of information and objects of work is visualized. For objectifying the ways of cooperation, Cooperation Pictures represent:

- places between which information and objects are exchanged;
- the kind of exchange (in the shape of annotated arrows) between places, which illustrates who passes on what entity or by what medium;
- errands to be performed by hospital staff and how patients make their way to the different units.

Construction process

Cooperation Pictures can be drawn after a series of interviews by the developers, and utilized for feedback in workshops with heterogeneous user groups. Due to the immediate understandability, they are also highly suitable for enabling user groups to develop Cooperation Pictures on their own during workshops, where the developers serve only as moderators.

Example

The illustration below shows the joint task "Admission of a Patient."

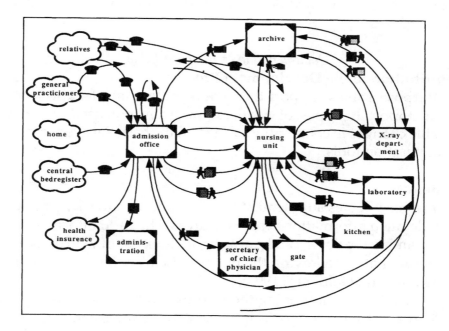

Project Experience

In our projects we were astonished about the usefulness of Cooperation Pictures. Due to the non-formal techniques of representation, users were able to immediately recognize themselves and their work within the used symbols and icons. The given "exercise" — visualizing a joint task — was clear. Without much time for explanation, they were able to actively participate in elaborating, discussing and introducing their activities, reasons for a particular task performance and necessary cooperation links to other departments. That means: Cooperation Pictures supply an appropriate subject of discussion which puts users directly into the position to reflect together about their own organization.

In our project context it was surprising for all workshop participants that within a regular admission of one patient in the morning; up to 17 phone calls are made and a series of errands are performed. Immediately a discussion about improving the process arose. Furthermore, for many users the wall painting manifested for the first time that their work does not consist in nursing a patient only, but that a not insignificant portion includes tasks for cooperation and documentation purposes.

Document Types Purpose Table
Contribution to the Development Process

Purpose Tables support the understanding and feedback of selected important types of cooperation. They are used to discuss possible changes in cooperation and form the basis for system design of cooperation tools.

Content

Purpose Tables supplement Cooperation Pictures by providing more detailed information at selected areas. They add information by:
- naming the objects at the arrows, in the sense of who does what, with what — following the pattern of Object Behavior Analysis (Rubin and Goldberg, 1992),
- additionally describing the purpose and implications of individual activities and objects in their cooperative context.

Construction Process

The sources to develop Purpose Tables are Scenarios, which capture the necessary details from the workplace perspective, and Cooperation Pictures for broad information from the organizational perspective.

Purpose Tables are developed by the designer team and revised with user groups during workshops.

Example

The example shows a Purpose Table of the "Registration for an X-Ray Examination."

Single Activities	Purpose/Implications
Physician writes the order on the physicians order form.	It is documented who ordered the test at what (forensic, quality assurance). To kick on the implementation of the test.
Physician puts the order entry sheet in the nurse's mail basket.	Nurse is alerted that she has to act. She knows what is planned with her patient.
Nurse enters patient's name, other relevant data and the type of test on the order entry sheet.	Nurse prepares the order entry sheet in order to relieve the physician of such burdens.
Nurse enters the test with pencil on the patient's flowsheet.	It is documented for every member of the care team and physicians when the examination was ordered and to which further examinations he is scheduled.
Nurse puts the order entry sheet in the physician's mail basket.	Physician knows that he has to validate the order.
Physician sees the order entry sheet in his basket, enters the relevant clinical information, signs it and puts it in the nurse's mail basket.	The physician that carries out the test knows what to do and that the ordering physician is responsible for the test.
Nurse carries the order entry sheet to the X-ray department.	The X-ray departement can schedule the test and the performing physician can check the order.
Radiology technician chooses a date for the test and conveys it by phone to the unit.	The tests are coordinated within the X-ray department. The nurses know when to take the patient to the X-ray Department..

Project Experience

In the scope of our project, we selected the registration for an X-ray examination as an example for an important cooperation type. Using the Purpose Tables it was discussed whether the present way of cooperation—requiring a signature from the physician for every X-ray registration — is sensible or whether it should be changed. In this case it was decided— deviating from other hospitals — to continue to require it. This was deemed necessary for reasons of quality assurance by the radiologists.

Having evaluated systems at the market, it needs to be noted that some of them neglect the cooperative parts of the task and only model the requirement "registration of an X-ray examination." It is presumed in those systems that the physician performs the registration by himself. Thus he writes a note for himself about which patients he has to register for an X-ray. With this note he goes to the computer and makes the required entries. Because he is now the only one responsible for registration, he won't enter the examination on the physician's order sheet. Thus any documentation of the ordering is omitted. Also the information for the nurse is lacking and thus the entry in the patient's flow sheet. Here it became evident to the users that systems cannot solely be chosen by their system functions. Rather, by making aware the additional purposes of tasks in respect to cooperation issues, they were able to estimate the implications of the systems for their specific work organization.

Document Type Task Pictures

Contribution to the Development Process

Task Pictures are used to receive feedback about the performance of tasks with user groups. They support the learning process concerning differences in the accomplishment of tasks at comparable workplaces of an organization (e.g., wards).

Content

A Task Picture describes the involved functional roles, the used material, and the kinds of interaction.

Construction process

For each Scenario a Task Pictures is prepared. User groups provide feedback and the pictures are revised.

Example

The example shows a Task Picture of "Accompanying and Documenting a Ward Round. "

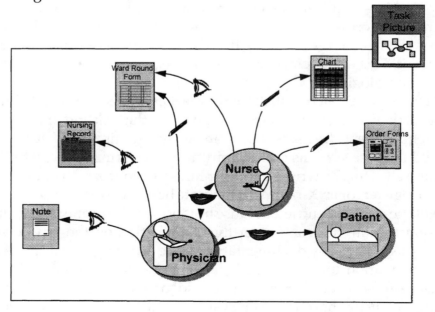

Project Experience

Similar to the usage of Cooperation Pictures, Task Pictures help in discussing the performance of tasks in an organization. Here, the subjects are not joint tasks across unit borders, but tasks being performed within one unit of a certain unit type from which there exist several units in an organization. In our project we recognized that by visualizing the tasks, we easily found out a lot of differences which otherwise would have been overlooked. The knowledge of possible differences led us into a position of clearly checking customization aspects of offered systems and elaborating concepts for customizable architectures.

Interim Summary: Analysis

Figure 1 provides an overview of the introduced document types and indicates the intended shift between the workplace and the organizational perspective. After each series of interviews, an understanding of the corresponding joint tasks can be achieved. On top of this a new series can be initiated. The successive evaluation of the developed Cooperation Pictures provides an increasing and profound understanding of the system requirements, and leads further to aspects of system design.

Figure 1: Document Types during Analysis

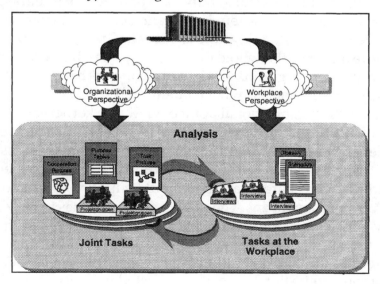

Design of the Future System Support

Parallel to the analysis of the current work practices, the determination of a task-oriented requirements specification along with discussions about design decisions need to take place. The gathering process for formulating requirements needs an on-going negotiation among the various user groups.

In the same manner as for the analysis of the current situation, a continuous shift is required between the organizational and workplace perspective. Here, we begin with the organizational perspective. It has to be first determined what major benefits the system should provide. Since hospitals (with their different and specialized units) have varying requirements, the future integrated system will be highly extensive. The resulting complexity can be handled by a useful subdivision with regard to certain characteristics. This necessitates agreement. For the means of reducing complexity and supporting negotiation processes, the document types Kernel System and System Stages are introduced.

The workplace perspective leads to the design of task support at the different workplaces. This is accomplished by applying System Visions and different kinds of Prototypes. Prototypes will be devoted to subjects such as tool support for types of cooperation, elaboration of group workplace support, and tools for single-task support.

To determine a useful subdivision of an entire integrated HIS, it is useful to identify a system kernel and separate it from specialized subsystems not belonging to the kernel. The application kernel is therefore a part of the whole integrated system. It is a sort of bracket supporting the integration and information flow between subsystems. For HIS it is still unclear what content the kernel should have.

From the organizational point of view, the kernel should support tasks of key units or departments which show a high cooperation profile. It has to satisfy urgent needs of the organization or tasks which are often performed. Additionally, it must support cooperation by providing main shared data and should supply a basic and uniform set of cooperation means. The application kernel has to be designed in a way which supports the integration of specialized systems. Out of these requirements, several technical requirements concerning the architecture and the openness of the system follows. The determination of the application kernel is manifested in a corresponding document.

Document Type Kernel System

Contribution to the Development Process

The document type Kernel System is used for reducing the complexity of the various and competing user requirements by defining the size of the system kernel.

It defines the kernel as a subset of the entire future integrated system which has to be implemented. It subdivides the kernel from specialized subsystems and defines interfaces to them.

Content

The document describes the extension of the application kernel and provides a graphical representation of the subdivision in a kernel and specialized subsystems.

Construction Process

The definition of the Kernel System is accomplished by developers on the basis of Cooperation Pictures and Scenarios. It is revised via input from user groups.

Example

The example presents an application kernel with subsystems for a hospital of small size:

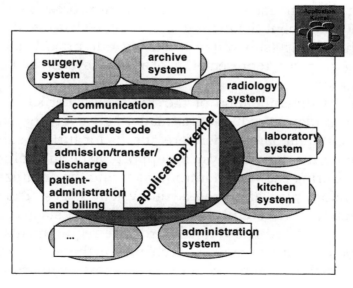

Project Experience

Out of our project experience, we definitely know that the design of integrated computer systems requires the involvement of heterogeneous user groups and the balance of their different interests. Each user group has its own profession and its own perspectives. Due to the differences in responsibility and tasks, these groups compete or are to a varying degree able to assert themselves against others. Each group is interested in an optimal support for its own work field whereas aspects of integration are less important. Also the time factor introduces additional pressure. Each domain wants to be autonomous and be served immediately (or first). Waiting for an integrated solution seems to be a less valuable goal. If they are no advocates for an integrated solution or they are not powerful enough, projects might undergo a severe crisis.

Therefore, the agreement on a kernel system is a major step in a HIS project. In our hospital, users and user management quickly grasped the idea of the application kernel with specialized systems being distinguished from it. Even in discussions outside the software project, they kept talking about the "application kernel." Since there are normally different possibilities for defining kernel systems, our example presents a solution for smaller hospitals. Large hospitals could use a kernel system for the clinical sections without the patient administration; they might use an integrated administration system capturing this functionality. The agreement process needs a lot of argumentation about the main integration needs as well as how to deal with existing (sub)systems. During our project, the easy-to-remember graphical representation of a kernel system helped us a lot in this process.

With the determination of the application kernel, a first step towards complexity reduction is made. However, the size of the kernel is still quite large. Therefore, it calls for further subdivision. Additionally, the degree of system support can be quite different and will grow during the system introduction into the organization. We must therefore plan and proceed in system stages. The resulting structure supports a careful planning of each of the stages concerning different aspects (e.g., additional hardware requirements, implications in the work task organization, changes in the environment, etc.). It also allows the planning and design of necessary interim solutions on different levels of detail. Their careful design can be very important in the acceptance of the total system.

Document Type System Stages

Contribution to the Development Process

System Stages support the subdivision of the still large application kernel. They determine the sequence of system development and introduction. They also build a foundation for System Visions and Prototypes for workplaces. Furthermore, System Stages enable the planning of interim solutions and the respective system requirements.

Content

System Stages determine the logical dependencies of the functionality of the application kernel. They describe within each stage the system support for tasks which are quite independent.

Construction Process

The System Stages are defined by developers on the basis of the document Kernel System, the Cooperation Pictures and the Scenarios. They capture both, the organizational and the workplace perspective.

Example

The example shows stages of the application kernel:

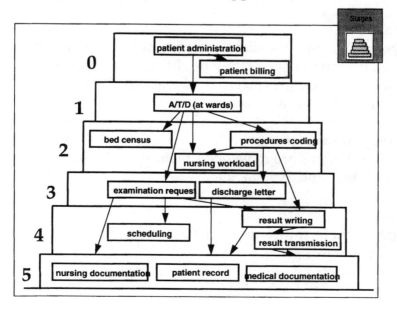

Project Experience

From our project experience we only can emphasize the usefulness of system stages. During a workshop at the end of the market analysis, we introduced concrete (named) stages for the system introduction. They made necessary sequences for system introduction transparent to the different user groups and the management. The neutrality of logical dependencies as reasons for certain unavoidable sequences helped accepting the order. We were astonished seeing one day after the workshop an information sheet covering the system stages being distributed across the whole hospital. Since then the concrete system stages have formed a part of our common project language.

To switch to a workplace perspective, we use means such as System Visions and Prototypes to facilitate the design and communication with future users.

Document Type System Visions

Contribution to the Development Process

System Visions describe the future system-supported performance of tasks. They relate Scenarios with Prototypes and show, therefore, the imbedding of the system in the environmental setting. They provide means for discussion among developers about the appearance of the system.

Content

System Visions describe the performance of selected tasks and anticipated system usage. They might focus on the performance of single tasks, the design of group workplaces or the accomplishment of cooperation and coordination.

Construction Process

System Visions are developed mainly on the basis of Scenarios, Purpose Tables and System Stages.

Example

The example shows parts of the System Vision "Design of the Ward Group Workplace."

The ward group workplace is subdivided in an information and a working area. Intention of the information area lies in providing overview information as well as hints about changes without being logged in. Aim of the working area is the provision of the proper work place with access to detailed information and the dealing with and sending of documents. The work place is accessible only by being logged in. Without anybody in the system the overview information ist shown.

The overview information includes ...

The switch between both areas is easily performed by ...

A quick log in and log out is supporte by ...

Project Experience

Cooperation support in hospital systems require innovative design ideas. As we recognized on the market during our project, there is still a lack of established ways to support certain kinds of cooperation being characteristic in hospitals. One topic is group workplaces at the ward. Using System Visions as outcome we tried to find useful concepts for system design. A leading force was to ask which of the already established ways of work organization which we identified at these places could be mirrored in a system and which of those could be redesigned because of new possibilities using the computer as media. The System Visions built the basis for constructing prototypes. Having shaped our own ideas with these prototypes, we were much more able to compare and evaluate the usage aspect of systems on the market.

Document Type Prototype

Contribution to the Development Process

Prototypes are developed with regard to the performance of single tasks, the arrangement of group workplaces, or the design of tools for cooperation support. They are used for illustration and feedback with users.

Content

Prototypes are operational models of selected aspects of the future system support.

Construction Process

Prototypes are oriented on System Visions.

Example

The example illustrates aspects of the design for group work-places: "Digest and Workplace of a Ward Group Workplace". The

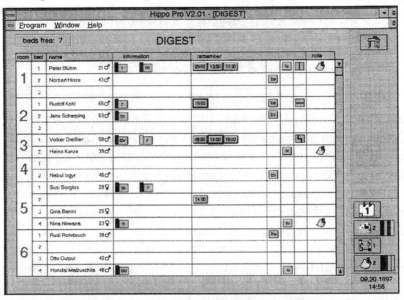

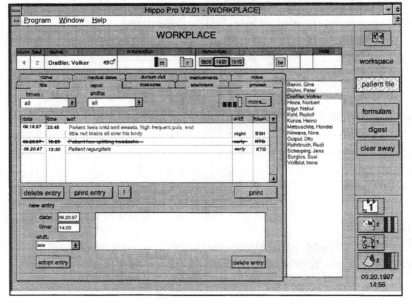

"design is according to the System Vision given above. You can see the digest (first screen dump) with overview over all patients and riders (forth column) giving information that changes in work tasks have occurred. Different colors of riders distinguish different shifts and professions (physicians and nurses). Additionally, valuable overview information, e.g., about the transportability of patients, their status, etc., are given. By clicking on the riders, you can jump directly into the opened patient record of the corresponding patient at the right page showing the new or changed description (second screen dump).

Project Experience

In our project we used the prototypes for working out criteria to measure existing systems according to their offered ergonomic and CSCW design. Since we built the prototypes in close cooperation with users, we found many useful ideas as well as detailed facts we could check and compare during system demonstrations on the market. Also users were promoted in understanding different concepts of system design for different functionality or cooperation support.

Interim Summary: Design

Figure 2 provides an overview of the introduced document types for supporting the task of systems requirements and design. Similar to method of proceeding during analysis of the current work situation, the choice of documents direct the intended shift between the organizational and workplace perspective. The document type System Stages reflects a special position which supports both perspectives.

Figure 2: Document Types During Design

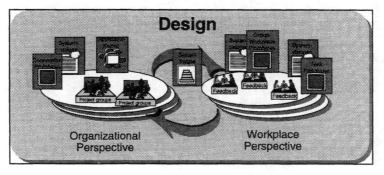

SUMMARY AND OUTLOOK

The presented approach directs a way to proceed in analysis and design of hospital information systems by providing easy-to-use document types. The recommended method with the four dimensions — switch between workplace and organizational perspective, user-oriented documents for supporting negotiation processes, close intertwining of analysis and design, and evolutionary proceeding — follows the three given guidelines for addressing different sources of complexity. The document types focus on different aspects of the complex cooperative work practices in different levels of detail, they support processes of agreement in a huge amount of competing requirements, and they provide means for discussing future system-supported work practice in comparison with the current organization. Figure 3 below provides a summary of the whole approach.

In the future we want to emphasize three further relevant aspects in the hospital domain. We investigate means for the customization process which demand extended ways to proceed during analysis, design and system adaptation. Secondly, we will focus on the role of groups (Grudin, 1994) as a third perspective beside the organizational and workplace point of view, along with all the necessary implications

Figure 3: Document Types During Analysis and Design

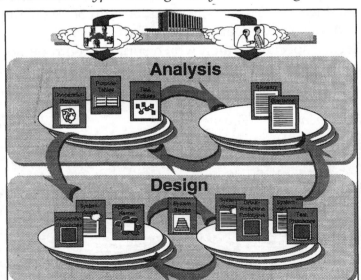

of our approach. Thirdly, we want to extend our experience with communicating (and documenting) project knowledge among developers and users by building-up WWW-based intranets providing templates and tools supporting the production of documents.

REFERENCES

Bürkle, U., Gryczan, G., &Züllighoven, H. (1995). Object-oriented System Development in a Banking Project: Methodology, Experience, and Conclusions. In: *Human-Computer-Interaction*, 10(2 & 3), 293-336.

Egger, E., & Wagner, I. (1993).Negotiating Temporal Orders. The Case of Collaborative Time Management in a Surgery Clinic. *CSCW: An International Journal*, 1(4), 255-276.

Floyd, C.(1987). Outline of a Paradigm Change in Software Engineering. In: G. Bjerknes, P. Ehn, M. Kyng (eds.): *Computer and Democracy*, Avebury, Gower Publishing Company Limited, Aldershot, 191-210.

Floyd, C., Reisin, F.-M., & Schmidt, G. (1989). STEPS to Software Development with Users. In: C. Ghezzi, J.A. McDermid (Hrsg.): *ESEC'89*, LNCS 387, Springer-Verlag, S. 48-64.

Floyd, C., Züllighoven, H., Budde, R., & Keil-Slawik, R. (Eds.). (1992). *Software Development and Reality Construction*. Springer Verlag, Berlin.

Grudin, J. (1994). Groupware and Social Dynamics: Eight Challenges for Developers. *Communications of the ACM*, 37(1), 92-105.

Krabbel, A., Ratuski, S., & Wetzel, I.(1996). Requirements Analysis of Joint Tasks in Hospitals. In: B. Dahlbom et al. (eds.): IRIS 19, Lokeberg, Sweden. *Gothenburg Studies in Informatics*, Report 8, 733-749.

Krabbel, A, Wetzel, I, S. & Ratuski:, S. (1996). Participation of Heterogeneous User Groups: Providing an Integrated Hospital Information System. In: J. Blomberg, F. Kensing, E. Dykstra-Erickson (Eds.): *PDC 96*, Cambridge, Massachusetts, 241-249.

Krabbel, A., Wetzel, I., & Züllighoven, H. (1997). On the Inevitable Intertwining of Analysis and Design: Developing Systems for Complex Cooperations, *Proceedings of the DIS 97*, Amsterdam, 205-213.

Malone, T.W., &Crowston, K. (1994). The Interdisciplinary Study of

Coordination. *ACM Computing Surveys*,26(1), 87-119.

Riehle, D., & Züllighoven, H. (1995) A Pattern Language for Tool Construction and Integration Based on the Tools and Materials Metaphor. In: J. O. Coplien, D. C. Schmidt (eds.): *Pattern Languages of Program Design*. Reading, Massachusetts: Addison-Wesley, 9-42.

Rubin, K.S., & Goldberg, A. (1992). Object Behaviour Analysis. In: *Communications of the ACM*, 35(9), 48-62.

Schmidt, K., & Bannon, L. (1992). Taking CSCW Seriously: Supporting Articulation Work. In: *Computer Supported Cooperative Work: An International Journal*, 1, 1–33.

Schneider, K., & Wagner, I. (1993). Constructing the 'Dossier Representatif'. Computer-Based Information-Sharing in French Hospitals. *CSCW: An International Journal*, 1(4), 229-254.

Simon, G., Long, K., & Ellis, J. (1996) The Coordination of Work Activities: Cooperation and Conflict in a Hospital Context, *CSCW: The Journal of Collaborative Computing*, 5, 1-31.

Suchman, L. (1995). Making Work Visible. In: *Communications of the ACM*, 38, 9, S. 56–64.

Wolf, C.G., & Karat, J. (1997). Capturing What is Needed in Multi-User System Design: Observations from the Design of Three Healthcare Systems, *Proceedings of the DIS 97*, Amsterdam, 405-415.

Chapter II

Healthcare Process Redesign: A Case Study

Minh Huynh and Sal Agnihothri
Binghamton University, USA

In this chapter, we present key principles and the limitations of business process reengineering (BPR) in general, and the use of BPR in healthcare in particular. We then present a case study of reengineering a healthcare process. The purpose of this case study is to explore the reality of how a BPR project is initiated, formulated, and implemented in a hospital setting and how it can fail. In the final discussion, we analyze the possible reasons for the failure of the BPR project and discuss their implication to the implementation of BPR in general.

INTRODUCTION

Designing or redesigning processes in order to produce outputs that meet organizational goals is one of the most important activities in any business. There have been enough discussions on this topic, which is commonly called business process reengineering (BPR), in the literature. In this chapter, we present key principles and the limitations of business process reengineering. We then briefly discuss the literature on the use of BPR in healthcare. Since information technology is one of the enablers of BPR, we also present the role of information systems and some useful technologies to capture information in healthcare. Finally, we present a case study of redesigning a healthcare process. The purpose of this case study is to explore the reality of how a BPR project is initiated, formulated, and implemented in a hospital setting and how it can fail. In the final discussion, we analyze the possible reasons for the failure of the BPR project and discuss their implication to the implementation of BPR in general.

PROCESS REDESIGN: PRELIMINARIES

Business process reengineering has been one of the hottest topics in management in the 1990s. There are several tutorials written on this topic including those by Grover and Malhotra (1997) and Rohleder and Silver (1997). The remarkable success of the best-seller book *Reengineering the Corporation: A Manifesto for Business Revolution* by Michael Hammer and James Champy (1993) is evidence of BPR's popularity. According to Hammer and Champy, "reengineering" is termed for the fundamental rethinking and radical redesign of business processes to achieve dramatic improvements in critical, contemporary measures of performance, such as cost, quality, service, and speed. Many executives (some surveys show that as many as 88% of large corporations) have initiated BPR projects as a way to turn their companies around, to regain their competitive edge, and eventually to boost their profitability.

Reengineering entails seven basic principles of doing work, relating to who does the work, where and when it is done, and information gathering and integration (Hammer, 1990). These principles are summarized below.

- *Organize around outcomes, not tasks.* Have one person or a team perform all the steps in a process. Design that person's job around an outcome instead of a single task. Organizing around outcomes eliminates the need for handoffs, resulting in greater speed, productivity and customer responsiveness. It also provides a single knowledgeable point of contact for the customer.
- *Have those who use the output of the process perform the process.* Instead of establishing specialized departments to handle specialized processes in order to benefit from specialization and scale, let the people closest to the process actually perform the work. Relocating the work in this fashion eliminates the need to coordinate the performers and users of a process.
- *Merge information-processing work into the real work that produces the*

information. People who collect information should also be responsible for processing it. This minimizes the need for another group to reconcile and process that information and reduces errors.

- *Treat geographically dispersed resources as though they were centralized*. Although decentralizing a resource improves flexibility and service, it gives rise to redundancy, bureaucracy, and missed economies of scale. Centralization could be achieved by using databases, telecommunications networks, and standardized processing systems.
- *Link parallel activities instead of integrating their results*. Forge links between parallel functions and coordinate them while their activities are in process, rather than after they are completed. Communications networks, shared databases, and teleconferencing could be used to achieve ongoing coordination.
- *Put the decision point where the work is performed, and build control into the process*. People who do the work should make the decisions. This way, it is possible to have a flattened organization with fewer layers of management and organizations that are more responsive.
- *Capture information once and at the source*. Today with on-line databases and Internet access, it is easy to collect and store the information simultaneously. Bar coding, relational databases, and electronic data interchange make it easy to collect, store and transmit information. This avoids erroneous data entries and costly reentries.

The critical reappraisal of BPR in itself is an interesting proposition. Despite the claims of the tremendous success in BPR as presented by Hammer and Champy, as well as other reengineering proponents, there exist problems within BPR approach. Many researchers have studied the actual practices of BPR in organizations and reported the lessons learned (for example, Caron et al., 1994; Stoddard & Jarvenpaa, 1995).

In 1993, a survey of more than 500 CIOs by Deloitte & Touche's Consulting Services reveals that although a growing number of CIOs are involved in reengineering projects, BPR projects usually bring with it big-time problems and very often failure. Even Michael Hammer, the guru of reengineering, admitted that most reengineering projects are fraught with problems and estimates as many as 70% of these projects are failing (Moad, 1993). Davenport and Stoddard (1994) identify, discuss, and dispel the reengineering myths. The survey in literature on the topic of BPR reveals a wide-range of possible causes that may contribute to the failure of BPR projects. Among those possible causes are the following:

- Reengineering function rather than process.
- Selecting wrong process to reengineer.
- Flawed study of the current situation.
- Lacking the detailed methodology to do reengineering.
- Reengineering under a constraint financial budget and insufficient staff resources.
- Use of available resources instead of investigating best resources.
- Ignoring the cost/benefit factor.
- Ignoring the existence of surrounding context.
- Ignoring the effect of changes on workers.
- Lacking inputs from those at the front lines of the process.
- Lack or insufficient communication with employees.
- Senior management not 100% supportive.
- Lack of coordination between IT and BPR.
- Including non-value-added processes in the BPR project.

Bashein, et al. (1994) discuss the organizational preconditions that set the stage for BPR success or failure. Based on the literature survey related to BPR, the conditions that can influence the outcome of a BPR project are summarized below.

- BPR project may not succeed when it relies solely on the use of information technology for the redesign of the process. Although the use of information technology is essential, it is not a sufficient condition for the success of creating a new process. A deeper understanding of the logic and structure under the current practices is required. This means BPR must take into account not just the technological choice but also the critical factor of human interaction embedded within the process.
- BPR project may not succeed when it relies solely on the top-down approach. The support and commitment from the management leadership is no doubt crucial in BPR, but these alone cannot successfully transform the process. It is important to make BPR acceptable and beneficial to users of the process. Hence, BPR

requires a strong participation and partnership from those at the front lines of the process. This means BPR must be established on an effective two-way communication between those at the top management and those closest to the process.

- BPR may not succeed when it is used to set unrealistic expectation. When management initiates BPR with a hope of solving a complex problem and trying to create major impact in a short time, the result is often disappointment. The reason lies in one of BPR's basic assumptions that to redesign process, one needs to throw away the existing process and start from scratch. This assumption ignores the existence of a surrounding context. Since none of the process can exist in a vacuum or by itself, process has to exist in a larger environment with which it must interact and by which it must be constrained. Hence, starting from scratch is just a costly illusion.

- BPR may not succeed when it focuses on the different way of doing the same thing rather than trying new things to meet new demands. BPR's narrow focus on just the process can be fatal, because in some cases changing the process may be the wrong way to solve the organization's problem. The case of Britannica is an example of how reengineering would be an inappropriate solution to the company's problem. In the age of multimedia, when a CD-ROM version of the encyclopedia has been developed and is widely available, reengineering production of the old paper-based encyclopedia will not help. The important point is that BPR should stress not just redesign, rethinking, but also reinventing the process to meet the dynamic changes in the business environment.

REENGINEERING IN HEALTHCARE

The healthcare industry is going through rapid changes because of the increased competition and changing relationships with the purchasers and payers. Because of this, there is a growing interest among hospitals to reengineer their processes. Walston and Kimberly (1997) claim that "over 60 percent of all U.S. hospitals are involved in reengineering initiatives" and that "literally billions of dollars are being spent in the name of reengineering." Bigelow (1998) critiqued the existing literature on reengineering and addresses the conundrum hospital executives encounter when faced with the decision to reengineer. She claims that although BPR promises big improvements, "so far there is little indication what impact reengineering has on hospital performance. Although the healthcare literature gives the impression that reengineering is as equally necessary and appropriate for hospitals as it is for private industry, no research is presented that studies reengineering's efficacy. The claims of success usually are mere announcements of goals and expectations, and the anecdotal evidence suggests that hospitals are not engaged in reengineering. Despite these limitations, prescriptive writings urge hospitals to undergo reengineering if they are to survive. She further argues that important assumptions underlying reengineering do not apply to hospitals. For example, the assumption that "reengineering begins with no assumptions and no givens...it ignores what is and concentrates on what should be" is not appropriate for hospitals. This assumption implies that hospitals have control over their services and practices, which often is not true. For example, hospitals can not add or delete services with the same freedom as most firms in private industry. Similarly, although the success or failure of reengineering depends on the top management's commitment, hospitals do not have much control over physicians, who can exert significant control over any attempts to fundamentally rethink the delivery of patient care in a hospital. Physicians provide much of the actual care and influence patient referrals, making them a key customer as well as a key member of a hospital's internal work processes. Gordon (1999) claims that instead of focusing on processes in order to improve patient satisfaction, too many hospitals continue to focus on technology, employees or marketing.

Since information technology is one of the enablers of BPR, we next present the role of information systems and some useful technologies to capture information in healthcare, before we explain the case study.

THE ROLE OF INFORMATION SYSTEMS IN HEALTHCARE

Information systems are no doubt an integral part of today's healthcare environment. Erica Drazen, vice-president at First Consulting Group, Boston, describes, "...The key tasks of managed care

are to identify best practices, coordinate physicians and other staff, ensure compliance with established clinical protocols and referral guidelines, and getting specialist feedback." All of these tasks are difficult to carry out when relying on personal memory or paper records alone. She admits, "You can't do all of those tasks if you don't have information systems support" (Appleby, 1996).

To understand the important role of healthcare information systems, we first need to realize the significant transformation that takes place in today's medical practice. The advent of advanced information technology has transformed many aspects of healthcare delivery processes. Information technology in many cases has functioned as an enabler to facilitate significant changes within a healthcare system, especially through the process of reengineering. Consequently, practicing medicine is increasingly relying on the processing, evaluation, synthesis, and transmission of information. There is a continuous need for healthcare practitioners to access, manage, and incorporate new information, new knowledge, and new capabilities into their practices.

In a typical day, a staggering amount of information flows between health care professionals and their patients, colleagues, ancillary service vendors (such as laboratories and home health agencies), knowledge resources, and purchasers (Schneider, et al., 1998). Today's information systems serve many functions in managing this flow of information. A well-designed system can inform doctors about treatment protocols and detect the potential drug reaction in advance. Based on the information that it stores, the system can alert physicians to whether a new prescription might interfere with existing drugs that the patient currently takes (Serb, 1998). This is just one example of how an information system can be designed and used for guiding the practice of medicine. In addition, physicians can use information systems to perform a host of other functions instantly. Information systems allow them to update their notes at any time and in any place. The systems can take order prescriptions from the doctors online. Through information systems, doctors can access patient's computerized records and view diagnostic images without waiting for the availability of the patient's paper chart. In essence, the computerization and communication links that are provided through information systems are the driving force behind many significant changes in today's medical practice. From all of these changes, we derive that the fundamental role of information systems is to provide healthcare practitioners the resources to manage their knowledge effectively and to share the available information efficiently.

To understand this important role of information systems in healthcare, it might be useful to distinguish different purposes that a system is designed for. Baldwin (1999) provides a useful way of categorizing six different levels of information systems used in healthcare. The six basic levels provide sufficient coverage of all the basic information needed in healthcare that involve clinical management, record storage & retrieval, and financial transaction management. Table 1 below shows Baldwin's six levels of system along with the actual system design and implementation that is associated with each of the levels.

This classification provides a useful context for understanding the case presented later. As we will point out, the order communication management systems (OCMS) are among the core system implementations that can drastically change many aspects of clinical activities and communication channels in a hospital. The OCMS can potentially offer rapid, efficient, and detailed communication links between physicians and ancillary service providers, e.g. laboratory, pharmacy, hospital, home health agency.

Table 1: Six Levels of Information Systems Used in Healthcare

Level of System	Focus of System	System Implementation
Level 6	Clinical outcomes, disease management	Clinical information systems
Level 5	Enterprise-wide data repository	Computerized patient records
Level 4	Point-of-care clinical charting	Computerized patient records
Level 3	Clinical orders applications	Order communication Management systems
Level 2	Ancillary department applications	Order communication Management systems, Computerized patient records
Level 1	Basic billing applications	Financial tracking systems

SOME USEFUL TECHNOLOGIES
TO GATHER INFORMATION

In the previous section, we identified information systems in healthcare as an important resource for knowledge management. The deployment of information systems is one of the key factors that enable many changes in healthcare practice. In this section, we present some of the essential technologies that empower these information systems. The emphasis here is not on the technical features of these technologies but on their potential for application in healthcare. We will highlight the benefits and limitations of these technologies from the experiences of those organizations that had used these technologies in the past. Although there is a wide range of technologies available, we choose to focus mainly on those technologies that are most promising to be useful for healthcare. These technologies include paging systems, wireless communications, voice-recognition applications, pen-based computing, intranet, Internet, Web applications, remote access, and document imaging systems.

Pager: The pager is a very good communication tool for doctors' use both inside and outside of the hospital. Today's pager can do much more than simply flashing the caller's telephone number. It can transmit not only telephone numbers but also entire text messages and other data. The promising feature in today's pager is its ability to communicate with a computer. Software available can send and receive messages up to 240 characters from a computer to a pager. Such a link can be expanded to two-way communication. With a pager, the doctors can be reached instantly when needed. The key advantage of the pager is that it helps to improve accessibility and to eliminate frustrating phone tag. With the system, a doctor can make his rounds of patient care anywhere in the building and still be in touch when necessary.

Wireless Technology: A number of wireless terminals have been developed for clinicians to carry with them to record data. The portable wireless terminals are usually light, tough, and easy to use. They also have big screen for display. The portable wireless terminals can be linked to a central computer via wireless LANs. Such LANs have been developed using the technology called "spread-spectrum" radio. Message transmitted using "spread-spectrum" radio is highly secure, because a single message is divided into many small pieces using a special code, and all of these pieces are sent over different frequencies. At the receiving end, the same code is needed to reassemble the message (Gardner, 1993).

Wireless terminals such as "Meditech," used at the JFK Medical Center in Atlantis, Florida, help to record patients' vital signs, input and output, and blood glucose levels. Others such as "Infolio," used at Stanford University Medical Center, serve as an "electronic clipboard" for checking off patients' information on the electronic forms. All of the information obtained from these wireless terminals can then be transmitted to the central system for further processing. Wireless communication devices have a potential to replace the traditional way of data collection with paper and pen at the hospital. Doctors can use it for direct order-entry without relying on any forms. Wireless communications offer a convenient but flexible medium for the automation of an order communication management system in a hospital.

Voice Technology: Voice technology is perhaps one of the most promising interfaces that can break the keyboard barrier and facilitate the labor-intensive task of data input. Despite its long-presence as a data input device, keyboard has many shortcomings. Unlike the keyboard, voice technology does not rely on typing. Through voice recognition, the input process is more natural, convenient, and much easier to use than the labor-intensive process of data input via the keyboard. In recent years, there have been a number of voice technology products available in the market. Some of them have been adapted for use in hospitals. One such product is LawTALK. It is one of the few systems that use voice input to interact with an on-line retrieval system. The system also provides interface with word processor programs such as WordPerfect. Voice technology has many benefits, including the following:
- It saves outside transcription costs.
- It provides more thorough documentation and hence reduces the risk of liability lawsuits.
- It helps to reduce time in documentation.
- It reduces the likelihood of forgetting important information.
- It improves the productivity of doctors who are PC phobic (Betts,

1994, p. 73).

Despite many of its potential uses and benefits, the present voice technology still has limitations. The most critical is that voice technology is more suitable for on-line input of data but not appropriate for output of information. Generally, the output is too voluminous to be retained by the average user. Furthermore, the eye can assimilate much more information in less time and quicker than the ear (Hawkins, 1994, p. 68). Finally, the use of voice technology often involves more than a replacement of keyboard. It requires the rethinking of tasks and redesign of work processes (Hilton, 1994, p. 33). Hence, if not implement properly, voice technology could hinder the process rather improve it.

Pen-Based Computing: Using a pen as an input device is natural, because everyone has used paper and pen before. There are two broad categories in pen-based computing system. The first kind is designed to manipulate on-screen graphic objects. A pen simply replaces a mouse for ease of movement and control. Using a pen rather than a mouse also helps to reduce the risk of repetitive stress injuries. The second kind is a pen-tablet system that supports handwriting and serves as replacement for both mouse and keyboard. However, handwriting recognition is still the weakest part of pen input. With the user's consistent training, the system can recognize up to 90% of his/her handwriting (Hilton, 1994, p. 33).

Many companies have succeeded in using pen-based computing systems to improve their work process. One of them was New Jersey Bell, which tried to automate field management with the aid of a pen-based computing system. The system enabled the company to use human resources more efficiently, cut down paper work, and reduce data redundancy (Kurelia & Young, 1994, p. 35). Another company making use of the pen-based system innovatively was Consolidated Rail Corp. The company combined the advantage of pen-based computers with the power of a communication network to create an on-line and mobile order processing system. The system helps improve the timely response to the customer's need by creating an on-line, mobile communication link between the crews and the staff. The results were the drastic increase in efficiency and productivity. For instance, the system enabled the train to get in and out of the plant much faster, to readjust its schedule and route to accommodate customers' need. With the use of pen-based computer, the delay and frustration caused by illegible orders were successfully eliminated (Lee, 1994, p. 30).

Network: Perhaps, one of the most dramatic recent developments in information technologies has been the fusion of computing and communications that led to the widespread use of the Internet. A recent survey by the Healthcare Information and Management Systems Society (HIMSS) show that 95% of respondents use the Internet compared to 87% in 1996 (Serb, 1998). Although healthcare systems have used the Internet mainly for business purposes, e.g. marketing, relaying e-mail, billing, and dealing with vendors and insurance companies, some of them start tapping into the Internet for clinical activities. For instance, the Internet has been used to relay patient records. It is also designed to allow patients to schedule their appointment online.

While healthcare may be slow in adopting the Internet, its usage of the intranet is much more widespread. The intranet allows organizations to use a private network to share records, make in-house referrals, and electronically sign reports. For instance, one Intranet based clinical system used at Scottsdale Healthcare in Arizona is able to distribute its diabetes management program electronically. Diabetics can send encrypted glucose readings to their doctors. Based on the results, the doctors can determine whether to see the patient or not. The doctors can also send back literature on the disease to the patient. All of these take place online via the intranet-based clinical system (Serb, 1998). One of the advantages of the intranet is its relatively secure environment. Information flow is protected by the control of a private network, which the Internet lacks as a result of its public nature.

The Internet and intranet are the driving force behind the design and implementation of Web-enabled systems that allow physicians to retrieve and analyze not only real-time patient data and diagnostic images, but also the patient's historical records from home and office. Such an integrated solution offers faster access to complete patient information as well as improved clinical decision-making (Odorisio, 1999).

Remote Access: In the advent of the Internet and the Intranet, remote access to diagnostic services is not only feasible but also strategically important. Of those surveyed by HIMSS, 27% say that remote access is a top driver of their information technology investments. Virtual access to information is essential because it provides doctors unique flexibility to work at any time and in any place. It has potential to save time and money, while increasing the healthcare quality and productivity. Remote access also makes it possible for physicians and clinicians to collaborate with each other, whether they are in the same building or miles away.

Most IT executives agree that remote access will be a big focus in the future because the healthcare organization is no longer defined by the campus and its services are no longer contained within a hospital's four walls.

Document Imaging System: The high-capacity physical media for storage of digital information, the increasing CPU power for processing of complex images, and the advancement in the imaging and workflow technology have underpinned the growth of document imaging systems. Given that multi-gigabyte disks and multi-processor CPUs are the norm on today's workstations, it is now feasible to create, store, process, transmit, and display sophisticated 3-D visualization of medical records. Computerized patient records become a reality.

American Management Systems (AMS) architects an enterprise-wide workflow and imaging solution in support of health information management (HIM), patient financial services (PFS), and human resources (HR) processes. These systems have completely revamped the ways business is conducted at Jewish Hospital Healthcare Services (JHHS), one of the adopters of AMS' workflow and imaging solution (Odorisio, 1999). The AMS's solution has eliminated the paper problem, saved record storage spaces, enhanced the productivity, and reduced labor costs. Most profound is the impact of the HIM system. Many headaches of the paper-based system have been eliminated as one physician user of the system commented, "...hours-long delays getting the old chart, lost medical records, charts lost, the need to store records off-campus, etc...no longer occur with electronic medical records" (Odorisio, 1999). Physicians are able to make better medical decisions with the system because they can access the patient records efficiently and timely from any where and at any time. The availability of the files for more than one person is a great advantage with the system. More importantly, the system is able to capture information more accurately, thus reducing unnecessary errors while increasing the efficiency.

A CASE STUDY

We now present a case in which BPR is applied in a project for the design, development, and implementation of a critical information system at a hospital. We will also discuss and analyze why BPR project at this organization failed to achieve its goals. Our objective is to demonstrate how the complexity in the process, the human interactions involved, and the existing technological infrastructure can affect the outcome of BPR and eventually reveal important limitations in the BPR approach.

The management of a local hospital, located at a rural community at the Northeast of the United States, was interested in a hospital-wide order communication management system (OCM) in order to improve its quality and performance. The objective of such a system is to communicate and process orders primarily from doctors efficiently. These orders are patient related and are related to, for example, tests, x-rays, medications, etc. At present, a paper-based order processing system is used like most other hospitals around the country. The problems caused by an inefficient ordering process will increase hospital and patient costs due to delays, errors, and waste of resources. To start the OCM plan, the management organized a working committee to guide the project. This committee consisted of a vice-president, a chief information officer, an administrator resident, a manager of nursing, a laboratory system coordinator, a radiology system coordinator, and an MIS coordinator. In addition to the hospital staff, a university team consisting of a doctoral student and a professor was also invited to serve on the committee as outsiders to facilitate and work on the project.

Because the OCM plan involved many complex processes, determining where to begin, what to do, and how to apply BPR turned out to be an enlightening task for the committee. The new OCM process would affect not only human interaction but also technology integration across different departments. The wide range of needs from various departments must be addressed; the diversity of orders within the hospital must be accommodated; and the different requirements in order-handling procedures must be satisfied. The effect of drastic changes would have a far-reaching repercussion in the way the hospital will operate in the future. Because of the complexity and the extensiveness in the proposed OCM plan, the BPR project conducted by the university team had to start with a process on a smaller and more manageable scale.

Define the Scope of the Study: With the time and resource constraints, the scope of the study was limited to West wing (WW) unit, one of the largest wings in the hospital. Because of the important role and the significant contribution of WW, the team found that WW is a good representative of the units in the hospital. Understanding the process in WW could provide valuable insights to the operation of other units in the hospital as well. Although work detail of WW could be different from other units, the overall procedures in ordering were very much similar among the units. Hence, the team predicted that any successful measures to improve the ordering process at WW would potentially be applicable and transferable to other units as well.

Understand the Current Process and Identify Problems: After specifying the objective of the study, the university team started to examine the current order processing system. Being outsiders to the hospital gave us an advantage of seeing things from an objective perspective. We looked at the process without worrying about the constraints and organizational politics. We first examined the ordering process at the WW unit. This unit was specialized in heart patients. One general manager was responsible for all the activities with the WW unit. The unit had a staff of 40 nurses and three unit clerks, and had 35 beds.

We interviewed the floor manager, nurses, unit clerks, and a doctor to learn about the order processing system, and observed the activities at the reception center where most of the activities occurred. We identified several problems related to the order processing at WW. Some of the major problems include poor scheduling, no standard procedure for getting things done, lack of coordination, and inefficiency of paper charting practice. We also gained a better understand of how an actual order was initiated, processed, and completed and identified several problems associated with the current process.

In addition to WW, we toured and interviewed personnel in two other departments which interact with WW very closely. The system coordinator of the first department shared with us her vision of an

OCM. According to her, the system should provide users at her department an on-line electronic access to the patient's record. From the system, the users should be able to view, retrieve, and update information related to the patient. Furthermore, the users should be able to look up the patient's chart and schedule for certain tests. She also mentioned three other features desirable in the new system. One, the system should be able to alert the users when the test is done and the result is available. Two, the system should be paperless so that there would be no more reliance on paper and forms for processing an order. Three, the system should provide a central link to all departments in the hospital so that order could be entered directly from anywhere and be processed online in a timely manner.

From our interview with the users in the second department, we learned that the basic requirements for an OCM system were similar to those at the first department. However, the system coordinator of the second department pointed out several specific enhancements that she wanted to incorporate in the new process. To reduce error, she would like information for orders to be captured at the source. The process should allow a unit clerk at each floor to enter their orders to the laboratory directly from the system. There should be no phone call or filling out of a paper form. She would like to enhance the current label using a bar code system. She was also interested in simplifying the order preparation and processing with more automation to reduce the training time.

From the WW unit's perspective, the system with scheduler was most desirable. The users wanted to access scheduling information and make decisions on a patient's daily activities chart so they could better plan their works. Also, a feature which allows direct order entry onto the system to bypass the paper and handwriting forms was desirable.

Develop Flowchart: The next task for the team was to translate the actual steps of the existing process into a flowchart. This required a deep understanding of the logic, structure, and information flow in the current process. The flowcharts were revised several times with comments from the people involved. The final flowchart helped us gain a broader perspective on the existing process, allowed us to locate possible process flaws and identify bottlenecks and non-value-added steps. It also helped us to come up with the measures of effectiveness for an order processing system. Finally, it gave us a foundation for the design of an ideal order processing system.

Collect Data: In order to substantiate the important contribution of WW and to justify our selection of WW as the site of the study, we collected data related to patient census. This included number of admissions, discharge, occupancy rate, length of stay, and patient days of both WW and the whole hospital. We then collected data on the volume of orders processed by both WW and by the whole hospital. This data gave us some evidence on the magnitude of the problem in the order processing system. By surveying the staff, we collected data to identify the root causes of the problem in the current order processing system. Using the survey, we also collected data related to the measures of effectiveness in an order processing system, which in turn would enable us to locate the flaws in the system, to recommend changes, and to assess the effect of implemented changes.

Analyze Data: The record of all inpatient procedures for the past data revealed that the hospital had processed an average of 95,000 orders per month. According to data collected on in-patients for a six-month period, WW contributed approximately 25% of all procedures processed in the hospital. It had more patients than any other units. The occupancy rate was between 80 and 90%. The duration of patient stay varied between three to five days. For the survey, we tabulated all the questionnaires completed by nurses, clerks, doctors, and patients. From the result of our survey, we were able to identify the following causes of the problems in the existing ordering process. They include illegible writing on the order, poor communication between doctors and nurses, poor scheduling, and errors and inconsistencies on the order.

According to our original plan, the next phase would involve the second round of data collection. This time we would focus on data relating to the root causes of the problem and on the measures of the effectiveness in the ordering process. We would design a check sheet for use in the data collection. The purpose of this data was to allow us to understand the impact of the current problems on the system. Using this, we also can measure the improvement when the processes are reengineered.

Meanwhile, we also started redesigning the process. The approach we took was to start with an ideal process, which was not subject to any organizational, budgetary, and technological constraints. A conceptual framework for the proposed ideal order processing system is explained in Figure 1. We then developed the ideal process into a flowchart that showed how an order was processed under a new system. We also explored the current and emerging

Figure 1: Conceptual Framework for the Proposal of an Ideal Order Processing System

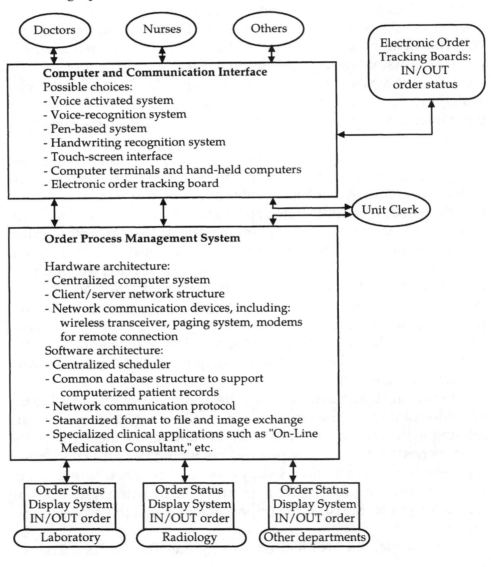

information technology to be incorporated into our ideal system. We searched for creative applications that are currently used at other sites or have potential use in the hospital environment.

As a first step in moving towards this ideal system, we suggested a simpler redesign, which considers the existing constraints. The revised system should overcome the flaws in the current manual-driven process. The approach is the automation of the current ordering process with the available information technology. The objectives are to eliminate the paperwork and to make use of a computerized scheduling system.

We presented our recommendations to the committee. Although the committee liked our recommendations, due to several occurrences within the organization including management restructure, the results of the study were not implemented and the project was postponed indefinitely.

LESSONS LEARNED AND CONCLUSION

One of the limitations of this project was the absence of two-way communication and the lack of partnership effort between the top-management and the front-line employees. First of all, the BPR project in this hospital was initiated without any strong sponsorship from the management. This is evident in the fact that no resources were committed or specifically allocated for the project. Although the leadership involved both the vice-president and CIO, their roles quickly disappeared soon after the project started. Secondly, the senior management did nothing to convey the BPR message and its importance to the employees. Most of the people with whom we came in contact had little idea what the OCM plan was. Each of them had different reactions to our BPR effort. On one occasion, a radiology system coordinator explicitly indicated that whatever the change was, they did not want to lose control of their systems. Thirdly, there was little participation in the project from people who were the actual users of the system or closest to the process. Neither doctors nor nurses served on the OCM committee. This perhaps attributed to the poor response rate from the doctors in our survey. In fact, when we received only one completed survey from the doctor, we could sense their negative attitude towards the overall OCM project. If doctors, who would be the ultimate users of the new OCM system, did not care and failed to participate in the project, the chance for acceptance of the new system would be slim.

The misleading information that we got from the MIS coordinator during our data-collection process provides an interesting insight of an internal conflict among key parties involved in the project. This is another indicator of poor communication and cooperation, which had to be resolved for the BPR project to be successful.

From these observations, it is logical for us to predict that when the BPR project has neither the support from the top management nor the participation from the front-line people, it will get little chance to succeed, as demonstrated in this case study.

When the OCM plan was first proposed, the vision was to build a system with central links to support the ordering processes throughout the hospital. BPR was the chosen approach, because the plan was directed toward the innovative use of information technology to support the hospital mission. However, as the study proceeded, the team realized that the actual ordering process was far more complex than expected. It was not a simple replacement of one system with another. When the logic and the structure of the current process was unveiled, the task of reengineering became monumental. First, there were issues related to human factors that must be resolved. For instance, the management needs to galvanize the support and cooperation from users such as doctors, nurses, system coordinators, etc. Secondly, there were existing technological infrastructures that must be integrated to the redesign. For instance, the management needs a strategy to analyze the cost/benefit issue involved, the disposition or reuse of the existing investments in computer systems, lab equipment, and other software applications at in both the laboratory and radiology. Simply abandoning all of previous investments may not be an attractive option. Hence, in a complex process, it is difficult to justify the decision of redesigning it from scratch. This additional evidence to disclaim the virtue of the "start with a clean sheet of paper" approach. In the case study, we also see a real-world situation in which a project is always facing constraints. For instance, there was a priority in budget allocation that restricted resources committed for the BPR project. When the priority was shifted, so were the resources. Hence, the change in resource support can have a drastic impact on the direction and momentum of the on-going project.

One of the methodological problems associated with this case study is the confusion in applying the BPR approach. When the process was too complex, we could not redesign the process directly. We had to first break the complex process into smaller and more manageable processes, then we focused on one of the smaller processes. Since we worked on the smaller process, we might not apply all the principles in BPR. In essence, we no longer did reengineering and hence we could achieve only an incremental change. This is contradictory to the fundamental objective of reengineering, which is to make radical changes.

In retrospect, we find that the organization was not ready for reengineering. It lacked management commitment. It did not have a strong leadership with a clear vision. It had no strategy in establishing two-way communication needed in the BPR. It could not get users such as doctors, nurses, and those on the front line to actively participate and provide input for the BPR initiative. The lack of management commitment was also evident in the fact that there was no funding to support the project. Basically, the management approached the project with an exploratory attitude. Their strategy was to incur neither cost nor risk in the proposal of a new system. As a result, the penalty for not implementing the proposed system was negligible. It would not be the case if a paid consultant was to conduct the study. Perhaps, then management would feel more committed toward the project.

Although there is a continued discussion on the appropriateness of reengineering in businesses, in our opinion it is very important to reevaluate and redesign business processes in order for the survival of the businesses in an ever-changing environment. However, the magnitude and frequency of the redesigning efforts may depend on the organizational constraints. Organizations need to understand these and take precautions before they reengineer processes so that they can avoid repeating some of the common mistakes. In addition, rapid changes in the information technologies provide many opportunities for reengineering processes successfully.

REFERENCES

Appleby, C. (1996, February 20). The mouse that roared. (better information technology needed for managed care). *Hospitals & Health Networks*, 70(4), 30-35.

Baldwin, G. (1999, March 22). Data systems may need some intensive care. *American Medical News*, 42(12), 27.

Bashein, B., Markus, L. M., & Riley, P. (1994) Preconditions for BPR Success. *Information Systems Management*, 11 (2), 7-13.

Bigelow, M.A. (1998). "Reengineering: Deja vu all over again," *Health Care Management Review*, 23(3), pp. 58-66.

Betts, M. (1994, June 27). Designing doctor-friendly systems a chore. *ComputerWorld*, 28(26), 73, 76.

Caron, R. J., Jarvenpaa, S. L., & Stoddard, D. B. (1994). Business Reengineering at CIGNA Corporation: Experiences and Lessons learned from the First five years. *MIS Quarterly*, 18 (3), 233.

Davenport, T. H. (1993) *Process Innovation: Reengineering Work through Information Technology*. Harvard Business School Press, Boston.

Davenport, T. H. & Stoddard, D. B. (1994). Reengineering: Business change of mythic proportions, *MIS Quarterly*, 18 (2), 121.

Gardner, E. (1993, April 5). Hospitals put wireless terminals to the test. *Modern Healthcare*, 23(14), 38.

Gordon, D. (1999). "Redefining processes to create a more humane patient environment," *Health Care Strategic Management*, 17 (3), pp. 14-16.

Grover, V. and Malhotra, M. (1997) "Business Process Reengineering: A tutorial on the concept, Evolution, Method, Technology and Application," *Journal of Operations Management*, 15, pp. 193-213.

Hammer, M. (1990, July-August). Reengineering Work: Don't Automate, Obliterate. *Harvard Business Review*.

Hammer, M. & Champy, J. (1993). *Reengineering the Corporation - A Manifesto for Business Revolution*, New York: Harper Business, a division of HarperCollins Publishers, Inc.

Hawkins, D. T. (1994, November-December). Breaking the keyboard barrier: Voice input to information retrieval system. *Online*, 18(6), 66-71.

Hilton, D. (1994, August). Alternate Input Devices Take a Load Off Wrists. *Managing Office Technology*, 39(8), 32-33.

Kurelia, T. & Young, D. (1994, January 1). The Pen is mightier Than the Mouse. *Telephone Engineer & Management*, 98(1), 34-35.

Lee, Yvonne L. (1994, February 28). Norand to release pen-based system with touch screen. *InfoWorld* 16 (9), 30.

Moad, J. (1993). Does reengineering really work? *Datamation*, 39(15), 22-28.

Odorisio, L. (1999, February). Imaging and Workflow. *Inform*, 13(2), 40-42.

Rohleder, T. and Silver, E. (1997). "A Tutorial on Business Process Improvement," *Journal of Operations Management*, 15, 139-154.

Schneider, R. & Eisenberg, J. (1998, May). Strategies and methods for aligning current and best medical practices: the role of information technologies. *The Western Journal of Medicine*, 168 (5), 311-317.

Serb, C. (1998, April 20). TechTravails. *Hospitals & Health Networks*, 72 (8), 39-41.

Stoddard, D. B. & Jarvenpaa, S L. (1995). Business Process Redesign: Tactics for managing Radical Change, *Journal of Management Information Systems*, 12 (1), 81.

Walston, S.L., and Kimberly, J.R. (1997). "Reengineering Hospitals: Evidence from the Field," *Hospitals and Health Services Administration*, 42(2), 143-63.

Chapter III

Information Security Framework for Health Information Systems

Lech J. Janczewski
The University of Auckland, New Zealand

This chapter outlines the major issues related to the security of medical information systems. Medical information systems are unique in this sense that integrity of the records and privacy issues are dominant. The presentation includes the formulation of the basic medical information security tenets as well as the discussion of the major components of the security subsystem: patient identification, access mechanism, reference monitor, communication subsystem and database subsystem. Also examples of privacy law are quoted and discussed.

Security is about the protection of assets. Information security deals with the protection of information within a given domain. In this context it is usually expanded into three different directions:

- **Confidentiality**
  Assurance that particular information is accessible (read, write, or execute) by authorised personnel only.
- **Integrity**
  Assurance that during processing no unauthorised changes of information are possible.
- **Availability**
  Assurance that information can be used at will.

The security of information within a medical information system is extremely important for a number of reasons:

- **Welfare of patients**
An innocent typing error: entering "+" instead of "-" (resulting in wrong information about an individual's blood group) could have deadly consequences! To say nothing of the social consequences, the financial cost of such errors could be devastating. Multimillion dollar court verdicts are not uncommon. The speed of accessing vital patient records is also important. In the emergency ward the surgery team could not afford a long wait for information about a patient's allergies.

- **Law enforced protection of patients' privacy**
In the majority of business world's disclosures of organisation secrets could have serious financial consequences, like lost transactions or clients. In the medical domain the situation is far more serious. Most countries have introduced law aimed at the protection of patients' privacy. Violations could lead to criminal court cases, usually being costly and lengthy.

- **Medical research requirements**
The law should protect the publication of case details, as was mentioned before, but medical information should be also available for researchers in the medical arena. Also, a significant number of medical personnel need to have access to patients files. Hence the characteristic dilemma of medical information: simultaneous needs for protection of data against disclosures with needs for its wide distribution.

The requirements of security of medical information systems could be contrasted with the security of military and banking systems as follows:

- In the military system confidentiality is usually the most important aspect of the security mechanisms (under no circumstances should our enemy know our plans).
- In the banking system, integrity of the data is usually most important (balance of the account reflects the reality of the performed transactions). Recent trends in banking indicate that availability is also becoming quite important. Twenty years ago cashing a cheque in a bank required many hours of waiting for

processing. Today's clients count the duration of processing of similar transactions in seconds.

- Most of the data stored within the system has a vital impact on patients' welfare. In view of this the integrity of the data is the most important problem. A small omission, such as a missing allergic agent, could result in the development of a life-threatening situation.

All that leads us to formulate the basic security tenets of medical information systems:

- **Every possible measure has to be introduced to limit the possibility of entering incorrect data or accidental changes of data**. Many countries have introduced parliamentary acts aimed at the protection of the privacy of individuals. These acts refer to the general public (Privacy Act – types) or to specific society groups, like patients (in the case of New Zealand: *The Health Information Privacy Act*, Privacy Commissioner, 1993). There are also relevant Codes of Ethics regarding medical practitioners, government officers, or others. On top of that there are customs regulating contact between patients and medical staff. These lead to the formulation of the next very important tenet of Health Information Network (HIN):

- **The system should adhere to all privacy requirements imposed by the law and customs of a country**. This is not as simple as it might look. Protection of privacy is quite important but the public interest is also of concern. Information about medical problems and treatments could be of great importance to the medical science (or society), and some parts of it should be available to medical staff and the public. Therefore another HIN tenet should be set up:

- **The Health Information Network system should protect the privacy of the individual but should limit that protection only to the information identifying the concerned individual and allow medical practitioners to use the data for their professional activities**. A medical researcher querying the system about various aspects of coronary disease is able to wait a relatively long period of time before getting the answer. By contrast, an emergency room team cannot wait hours for confirmation of a patient's blood group. This is the base of the final HIN tenet:

- **The Health Information Network response time (and therefore; availability) should be matched with the possible expectations of it users.**

Let us discuss a number of issues related to the security tenets of medical information systems. One of the most important is the question of the protection of patient privacy.

ISSUE OF PRIVACY PROTECTION IN THE MEDICAL INFORMATION SYSTEMS

In many cases, arguments have been made about breaching privacy for the good of the individual or for the good of society. Who is to define the boundaries of such good? At this point let us consider two entities: the *individual* and the *society*. We may assume that there is a continuum between the two entities concerning their view of privacy issues. Each entity could have a different point of view. We may say that *privacy* has the meaning of a point on this continuum.

The Privacy position is in fact a function of at least three variables: the Society as a whole, the individual concerned and some other

Figure 1: Privacy Continuum

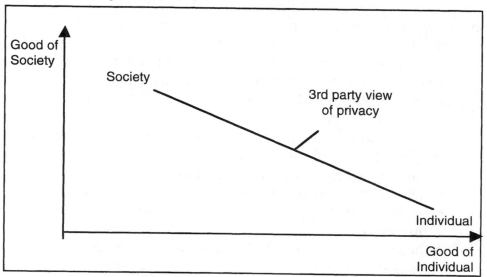

members of society. It is illustrated in the Figure 1 (adopted from Keng, 1998). Most of the existing legal frameworks try to compromise these conflicting points of view.

As it was said in the introduction, security issues in medical information systems are supported by many recommendations like parliamentary acts or standards. The practical solutions could vary from country to country and are subject to rapid change. In this chapter a New Zealand example will be presented. It is was chosen for the following reasons:

- The privacy protection mechanisms set up in New Zealand were based on international recommendations.
- The development procedure took into consideration the existing local solution and customs.
- The basic structure was set up several years ago which allows a critical point of view based on facts rather than of researchers' bias.

The list of acts related to data security issues introduced by the New Zealand Parliament is quite long. The following acts should be mentioned (Longworth, 1995): Trademarks Act 1953, Designs Act 1953, Patents Act 1953, Crimes Act 1961, Copyright Act 1962, Whanganui Computer Centre Act 1976, Evidence Amendment Act 1980, Official Information Act 1982, Privacy Commissioner Act 1991, and Privacy Act 1993. The most important of them is the Privacy Act. The Privacy Act not only fulfils the OECD (1988) statements, but goes beyond them through formulating 12 so-called "Information Privacy Principles" (Privacy Commissioner, 1993):

1. Personal information is only to be collected for a lawful purpose connected with a function or activity of the agency.
2. Information should be collected directly from the individual concerned.
3. The individual concerned should be aware that information is being collected and should know:
   - the purpose for which the information is being collected;
   - who are the intended recipients of the information;
   - the consequences for the individual if the information is not provided;
   - the rights of access to and correction of personal information

provided.

4. Personal information shall not be collected by unlawful or unfair or intrusive means.

5. Information is protected by security safeguards against loss, unauthorised access, use, disclosure or modification.

6. The individual concerned shall be entitled to obtain confirmation that information is held and access to information held.

7. The individual concerned shall be entitled to request correction, or a statement that such a change request has been made, to information held.

8. The holder of personal information must check its accuracy before use.

9. The holder of personal information may not keep that information for longer than necessary.

10. Information may only be used for the purpose for which it was originally intended.

11. The Holder of personal information may not disclose that information to any other person or agency.

12. The Holder of personal information may not assign a unique identity (key) unless it is necessary to carry out its function, nor may that identifier be that already used by another Holder.

New Zealand has an extensive social-support system. Over 10% of the workforce are receiving unemployment benefits. On the other hand, there is no nationwide method of identifying individuals. Social Security numbers are given only to those receiving social benefits; there are no nationwide internal passports or cards, even driving licences are without photos. Only recently (first quarter of 1999), after lengthy discussion new driving licenses with photos have been introduced. In view of the low level of criminal activity, this is perhaps justified, but the public is aware that violations of the social welfare system are frequent (e.g., welfare payments to persons not eligible for social benefits). Nevertheless the Wanganui Computer Act did not allow government departments to match their corresponding records. The Privacy Act 1993 incorporated the Wanganui Computer Act and the Privacy Commissioner Act plus OECD guidelines about data privacy (OECD, 1992). It allowed the matching of Inland Revenue, Social Security and Customs Department records — everything under the control of the Privacy Commissioner.

During 1998 the Privacy Act was under revision and a number of suggestions has been made aimed at making the spirit of the Act as clear as possible because in the past a lot of restrictions were wrongly interpreted and implemented (Privacy Commissioner, 1998).

A year after the introduction of the Privacy Act, a similar act regulating privacy issues in the medical sector (Privacy Commissioner, 1994) was introduced. Basically it elaborates in a more detailed way the interpretation of the 12 Privacy Principles set up by the Privacy Act 1993.

After eight years of existence, in the opinion of the author, the privacy protection legislation in New Zealand could be assessed as follows:

- Basic privacy protection is well developed.
- The office of the Privacy Commissioner is doing a good job, but due to limited resources and resulting small staff, is very slow in investigating the complaints.
- These delays could be a source of significant problems in the future, as several countries have introduced a law forbidding the export of data to countries lacking proper data protection and New Zealand could be considered to belong to such a group of countries.
- Public awareness of the possible lack of protection of privacy is very high, but at the same time is lacking in substance. There are numerous examples indicating that there are misconceptions as to what are the privileges and duties of the Privacy Commissioner Office.

GENERIC MEDICAL INFORMATION SYSTEM

Discussion of the security features in a medical information system requires the definition of what usually comprises a typical information system in such an environment. Figure 2 (adopted from Janczewski/Singh, 1998) gives an example of such installation.

Of course the reality could be dramatically different but some common features must exist as indicated in Figure 2:

- Connection to the supervising authorities; local or national (federal).
- Some information services could be outsourced. These services could be shared with other medical institutions.

- The hospital LAN should service most of the PCs and provide selective access to such subsystems as the administration of the facilities, payroll, nurses' roster, etc.
- Contact with the outside world should be provided by a dedicated mail system.

Figure 2: System Architecture of Typical Hospital

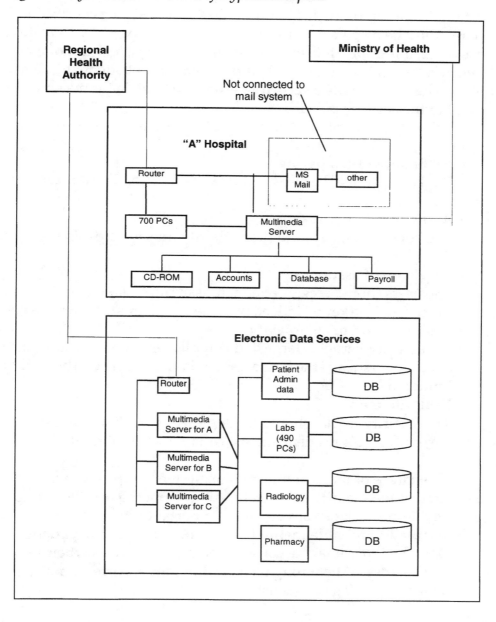

PARAMETERS OF THE SECURITY SUBSYSTEM

All the security requirements mentioned so far should be enforced by the implementation of security measures being of the hardware, software and organisational nature. Theoretically with the rational creation of medical information systems, the security functions could be dispersed between the system components. In reality, however, it is impossible to achieve this as security features of many legacy subsystems as off-the-shelf products are not adequate. Hence we are forced to create a **security kernel** responsible for the enforcement of the security policies.

The most important parameters of the kernel should be (after Amoroso, 1994):

- **Avoidance of tampering**
  The kernel should be resistant to malicious or inadvertent tampering.
- **Avoidance of bypassing**
  The kernel design should preclude attempts to access the system "around" the kernel.
- **Provision of assurance**
  The users should receive adequate assurance that the design and function of the kernel indeed provide an adequate security level.
- **Minimisation of complexity**
  If a security kernel is large and complicated, then the assurance procedures such as the formal methods and testing will be greatly hindered.
- **Fault tolerance**
  The security kernel should be designed in such a manner as to ensure that it is resilient against certain classes of faults.

The nature of medical information systems imposes several parameters of the security subsystem. Apart from the need to set up a security kernel other issues are quite important:

- **Simple but reliable method of identification of the patient**
  One can easily imagine consequences of a situation when somebody accessed the wrong file and provided incorrect data about patients' hearing problems!

- **Reliable method of identifying and authenticating the user of the system**

  This is a very important problem, as the unauthorised leak of data might have substantial consequences to the administration, including negative exposure and financial losses (through court actions). Also, the hospital environment is changing rapidly and today's access authority may not be valid tomorrow.

- **Medical data may be of any possible format: plain text, pictures, video, sound.**

  In the past the medical information systems tend to concentrate on processing textual information only. Development of the mass storage technology now allows storage and retrieval of multimedia information.

- **Extent of using cryptography**

  Most of the medical data is almost useless (except for researchers) if is not attached to a specific person. Hence, in the opinion of the author, encryption of all patients' data is generally not needed. Numbers (not the patients' IDs) could identify medical records, and only the association between these numbers and patient plus patient basic records should be encrypted. Basic patient data means such information as name, date of birth, address, financial status, etc. Of course inference attacks are always possible and by clever reasoning one might identify somebody's medical records. Inference attacks will be discussed later in the text. However, the range of such disclosure would be fairly limited. Even if the perpetrator could identify somebody's specific test results the rest of the patient record would be still hidden, protected by the unique identifier of the test. Generally, privacy law and similar acts require the introduction of a "reasonable protection" of patient records, and 100% security is neither required nor possible.

- **Importance of the security of the telecommunication and database subsystems**

  Medical facilities are generally dispersed (physically). Usual practice is that each facility maintains its own database. This implies the usage of sophisticated communication facilities. A mechanism must be set up to control all these dispersed databases and communications channels assuring an adequate level of reliability and security.

In the text so far we have discussed the major requirements for the security system of medical information systems. In the next part we will look closely at the most important parts of the security system:

- Patient identification
- Access mechanism
- Reference monitor
- Communication subsystem
- Database subsystem

PATIENT IDENTIFICATION

The issue of patient identification is much more complex than it looks. The ultimate goal is to identify every patient within the system in a reliable, quick and affordable way. There are number of way of doing so:

- **Name of the patient as a patient ID**

  In Auckland, New Zealand, in the telephone directory there are 17 columns of the names "Jones," and among them 16 entries are described as "Jones J." Much worse situations exists in such cities as Singapore or Hong Kong where the names like "Liu" or "Li" occupy tens of pages. Hence the name of a patient should be used only as a secondary identifying parameter.

- **Social security number or similar number as a patient ID**

  This seems to be a perfect solution as these type of numbers are already in use in the majority of countries and could be easily expanded to cover the medical area. Unfortunately, it is not generally possible as the result of society's attitude towards the creation of centralised files on individuals (So called "Big Brother Watching" syndrome). Following these fears some countries introduced legislation explicitly outlawing such solutions. The cited before New Zealand Privacy Principle 12 refers directly to these situations.

- **Physical patient features as a patient ID**

  Information technology allows wide implementation of such technologies as finger scan or retina scan. These technologies will be discussed later in the text. Even such drastic solutions as planting microchips in the patient bodies are possible, from the technology and costing point of view. Again, at present, due to the social pressure, such solutions are not possible.

All that leads us to the conclusion that the best technical solution, which is the most socially acceptable, would be the introduction of numbers similar to the numbers used by credit card companies and used by patients in a similar way. As a matter of fact, many hospitals or insuring companies are acting this way already. The immediate question is to what extent such a card could be a source of identification. One can easily imagine a situation where a person for some reasons could not present his/her card. The consequences might be negligible or could lead to a tragedy or crime.

ACCESS MECHANISMS

Each user of a medical information system before being granted access to the information resources must undergo the procedure of identification and authentication. Identification is the procedures and mechanisms that allow agents external to a computer system to notify the system about their identity. Authentication is the procedures and mechanisms that allow a computer system to ensure that the stated identity of an external agent is correct. In a typical situation an agent types in a login and a password. The login is usually in the public domain, but the password is known only to the agent, or to the agent and system operator.

In a more general case, identification and authentication could be performed in many different ways. This is usually a function of available budget and required security. Also these operations must be as unobtrusive as possible. If the procedure of identification and authentication is long and complicated, the users will go to every length to disable the system. The identification and authentication procedures could be one of three categories. The access could be provided upon demonstration of:

- Something possessed (magnetic key, smart card),
- Something known (password, personal knowledge or associations),
- Physical characteristic (finger tips, weight, fingers' lengths, retina, voice print) ora combination of these.

It is also common practice to introduce a number of passwords guarding resources of different sensitivity or a system generating a one-off password. A set of passwords works in such a way that the user, after introduction to the lowest security domain, is challenged to provide a different password to access the more secure region, etc. This means that the user must remember a set of passwords and relate them to a particular security region.

Among the most powerful are the systems using a one-off password, i.e., a password that is used only once. Figure 3 presents the logic of such a system. It works in the following way. Each system user has a password generator in the form of a plastic card-size calculator. Inside the calculator there is a microchip which performs all the necessary calculations. When the user would like to get access to the system, he/she would switch on the card and enter his/her password. In response the calculator shows a number —the "challenge." At the same time the user would login to his/her computer system (using his/her login). If everything is working properly, the system should generate the same challenge number as the one generated by the card. A difference indicates that the system and the card have lost synchronisation due to some reason, such as unauthorised entry to the system or the use of the calculator in the meantime. However, if there is no difference then the operator may generate a "response" to the

Figure 3: One-off Password System

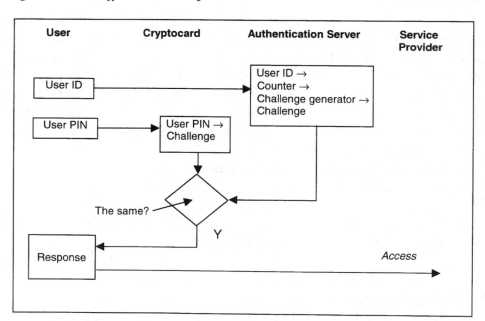

challenge on the card and enter it into the system. The system repeats the same calculations, and if it gets the same response, then the authenticity of the person is verified. This system offers a high degree of security but is a bit cumbersome in everyday, frequent use. It could be used for very sensitive medical systems.

In the present hospital environment, the most common method of accessing the system is by typing a login/password or using a magnetic card. Both methods do not offer a high degree of security. Typing in the login and password takes some time and could be recorded by third parties (by watching the operator). A magnetic card could be stolen or passed to an unauthorised person. At this stage of technology, the best solution seems to be using the finger scan technique. The scanners are the size of the computer mouse, and the scan takes a fraction of a second (Figure 4). Such devices cost about $100 and are easy to install and run. As identification is unique tampering with a finger scan device is significantly more difficult than with other identification and authentication devices.

An alternative method of identification and authentication of a system user could be the issuing of badges with a magnetic strip and a photo of the user. Such cards should work in conjunction with a personalised pin number.

At this moment there is a need to comment about identification methods based on items system users should posses and use to get access to the medical systems.

The widespread use of medical information systems around a nation could easily turn such items into a sort of recognised internal passport or ID card. This is what has happened with driving licences

Figure 4: Finger Scan Device

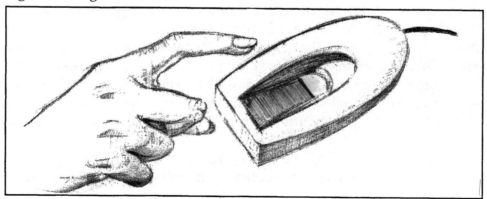

in many countries. This fact is exploited by many social groups claiming rightly or wrongly that the creation of such documents would make easier control of the population by the government and other agencies ("Big Brother Watching" syndrome). In many countries social pressure may practically prevent the introduction of such documents (e.g., New Zealand), while in the others such a document would be easily acceptable (e.g., Japan). On top of the social issues are managerial and economical problems related to the introduction and running of the ID system. In the opinion of the author, the finger scan system seems to be preferable as it reduces the mentioned syndrome worries as well saving a lot of the expenses relating to the reissue of lost or mutilated cards (fingertip patterns do not change throughout life).

REFERENCE MONITOR

Reference monitor is that part of the system that actually decides what kind of access could be granted to a particular system user. For instance, Dr. Smith should have access to all patient files while Nurse Brown only has access to her ward and only in the "read" mode. Before discussing the details of the reference monitor, we must comment about the general way these access privileges could be administered and what rules should apply in granting them.

Access control models can be classified as either Mandatory Access Control (MAC) or Discretionary Access Control (DAC). MAC is done through the comparison of the particular individual's clearance/authorisation to access the information with the classification/sensitivity, designation of the information, plus the form of access being mediated. Mandatory policies either require or can be satisfied by systems that can enforce a partial ordering of designations, namely, the designations must form a lattice. In the other words MAC means that within a system there is a central facility controlling all the accesses of all the users. DAC is the principal type of access control available in computer systems today. The basis of this kind of security is that an individual user, or program operating on his behalf, is allowed to specify explicitly the types of access other users have to information under his control.

Either MAC or DAC must be governed by the general rules of getting an access to resources policy. In hospital information systems the measure to protect against information misuse on a technical level is the controlling of data access of hospital staff according to the need-to-know principle. As stated in Holbein and Teufel (1995), need-to-know access controls reduce the information misuse risk because they ensure that an intended purpose exists when data access is granted. However, they do not prevent information misuse at all because a user's overall access context is not restricted to his/her current task within an organisation. A hospital is considered to be an ever-changing environment (users are changing, doctors and nurses come and go, policies change, etc). Thus, the access control model must also be flexible enough to support such a dynamic environment. The Role-Based Access Control (RBAC) seems to be the most appropriate for such conditions. The central tenet of the RBAC is that users do not have discretionary access to enterprise objects. Instead, access permission is administratively associated with roles, and users are administratively made members of appropriate roles. This idea greatly simplifies management of authorisation while providing an opportunity for greater flexibility in specifying and enforcing enterprise-specific protection policies. The other strengths of the RBAC model (Nyanchama/Osborn, 1994) are:

- The ability of enforcing the Principle of Least Privilege (RBAC's equivalent of "need-to-know" principle).
- Simplification of the complexity of system privilege management.
- Incorporation of application-level security constraints and semantics.

Finally, it is assumed that within the hospital information system it is possible to create the Trusted Computing Base (TCB) which contains all of the elements of the system responsible for supporting the security policy and supporting the isolation of objects (code and data) on which the protection is based. The bounds of the TCB equate to the "security perimeter" referenced in some computer security literature or the security kernel defined previously. For general-purpose systems, the TCB will include key elements of the operating system and may include all of the operating system. For embedded systems, the security policy may deal with objects in a way that is meaningful at the application level rather than at the operating systems level. Thus, the protection policy may be enforced in the application software rather than in the underlying operating system. The TCB will necessarily include all those portions of the operating system and application software essential to the support of the policy.

Following is the list of input elements that are the building blocks of a reference monitor for a typical hospital (Janczewski/Lo, 1998):

- **Primary Data Objects**
  These objects constitute the make up of the information stored in the hospital IS. Primary Data Objects fall into the groups of "Medical Information" (being items like: Diagnosis, Examination Request, Examination Results, Treatment Data) and "Non-Medical Information" (like: Administrative, Social, Personal Demographic, Insurance, Billing, etc.).

- **User Roles**
  These are roles that exist in the hospital. The example roles (after Pangalos, et al., 1995), are: Head Doctor, Responsible Doctor or Therapist, On Duty Doctor, Head Nurse, Nurse, Paramedical Staff, Paramedical Doctor, Registration Staff and Financial Staff.

- **Information Flow**
  This is the flow of information between users restricted by hospital rules and procedures in terms of identification and authentication. For instance a flow of information could be triggered by a visit of a patient to his/her GP. Starting from the initial registration, followed by record of the interview, diagnosis, referral to a hospital, admission to the hospital, request for additional tests, record of treatment, record of discharge, financial matters, etc.

- **System Architecture**
  This is the description of the system architecture. One may start from the layout of system components as it has been presented in Figure 2 and then follow with the detailed description of all the hardware and software components.

- **Class Hierarchy**
  This provides a representation of the relationship between the above mentioned objects.

The reference monitor usually consists of five logically independent components (enforced by separation kernel), being Object Manager (OM), Access Enforcement Facility (AEF), Access Decision Facility (ADF), Authorisation Control Enforcement Facility (ACEF) and Authorisation Control Decision Facility (ACDF). The ADF itself includes Ordinary Decision Engine (ODE), Exceptions Handling Decision Engine (EHDE), Security Metadata (SM), and Agents.

- **Object Manager**

  A multimedia server will most likely be built on top of an object-oriented database. It is therefore necessary to look at data in the server in terms of objects. The object manger involves creating, deleting, and updating multimedia objects and security objects. In an object-oriented environment, everything is considered to be an object with security attributes assigned to it. The object manager therefore will need to provide labelling functions for such classes of objects as Data Objects, Roles, Subjects, Interfaces, Transactions and Individual Accesses. The labelling must be consistent across all hospitals to allow inter-hospital reference validation. Looking at multimedia objects, a patient record is composed of medical and nonmedical data. In a multimedia environment, the Patient Record can be described as a "collection node," consisting of links pointing to various types of information (components). From this, it can be seen that there is a need for multilevel protection of the patient records. That is, only authorised users can access a particular type of hypermedia object.

- **ADF, AEF, ACEF and ACDF**

  The Access Decision Facility (ADF) is the essential part of the monitor. It is responsible for deciding whether a particular access is authorised and in what mode. For instance if Doctor Alexander is allowed to change the record of patient Rouse. The Access Enforcement Facility (AEF) is responsible for enforcement of activities in the target systems such that only permitted activities can happen in the target system. Furthermore the ADF itself is also treated as a target system and is administered by the Authorisation Control Enforcement Facility (ACEF) and Authorisation Control Decision Facility (ACDF) to determine whether an authorisation is authorised or not.

- **Ordinary Decision Engine**

  The ODE is part of the ADF and is responsible for determining whether or not the users' requests are authorised. The decision will be based on the RBAC and DAC rules stored in the Security Metadata. Generally speaking, the ODE will first determine the identity of the users by examining the *user id* in the request. It will then examine the required *access modes* to the particular objects and compare that with the access rights stored in the capability lists in the agents. As well as controlling individual accesses, the ODE also needs to control access on a higher level of granularity, namely, controlling user interface formatting and the authorisation of transactions. When requests are accepted, the ODE will inform the AEF to enforce such decisions by either allowing or disallowing the particular operations on the HTML pages.

When an agent becomes active in the multimedia server, identification and authentication processes will be undertaken and the user's role would be identified. From then on, the first task the ODE performs is to format the user interface according to the user's role. By user interface, we mean the multimedia page that the user can view. That is, layout of the pages, the structure of the pages (or collection). Furthermore, it will include functions (or transactions) that can be operated on the pages.

- **Security Metadata (SM)**

   The Security Metadata is the storage of the decision rules or metadata (like RBAC and DAC rules) for the ODE and EHDE. These rules are stored in a database which needs to be updated frequently; when situations such as when a new user is registered, a new patient record is created, a new role is introduced, etc. Furthermore, each time the SM is updated, it needs to resolve for conflicting roles (e.g., a person may not be a financial staff monitor and a nurse at the same time) to avoid a conflict of interests. Thus, there will be a need to store all possible conflict role combinations and each time a new role is created, updated, deleted, etc, conflicting roles are checked.

   There are two types of mechanisms available for the RBAC and DAC models, namely *capability list* and *access control list*. Capability list is used to centralise the access control validation process. The population of the capability list of agents will be accomplished by referring back to access control lists of the data objects. Actual rules would be stored in an access control list of the objects. An access control list involves the placement of a list of accessible subjects in each of the objects involved. Thus an access control list can be placed in each of the individual virtual patient records specifying the accessible roles for each of the records.

- **Exceptions Handling Decision Engine (EHDE)**

   If for any reason a request of an agent whose user's role is of critical importance (e.g. doctor on duty) is denied, the EHDE will take over the authorisation of the request. This is necessary because there may be some special circumstances where the access of information is needed but the user does not have explicit access rights. This action can be done in two ways: The first method is to have the head doctor (or someone in high authority) handle those exceptional situations with the ability to grant/revoke access rights. The person(s) will need to be trusted and always available. The second method is to have exception rules made for all possible situations. Thus in special situations, the EHDE will make a decision based on special rules such as "If the location of the terminal is in the operation room and the particular patient is in the hospital and another staff can confirm the need to access the information, then access is accepted." The system should have an audit control to validate the reason why there was a need to override the system.

Prediction of all the possible emergency situations is almost impossible and, for the simplicity of the system, it is better to use the first approach.

The basic components of the reference monitor are depicted in the Figure 5.

DATA COMMUNICATION SUBSYSTEM

The developments in the field of medical information systems let us formulate the following comments:

- Hospitals are building and running quite extensive information systems. These systems allows effective implementation and managing of quite complex databases.
- Most of the data traffic is between divisions of the same hospital, like sending X-ray results from the Radiology Department to a hospital ward.
- Exchange with the outside world is limited to the obligatory transfer of data required by the law or with some practitioners and laboratories cooperating with a hospital. Due to the protection of privacy and other laws, hospitals are reluctant to be engaged in a wider exchange of data.
- Despite fairly limited transfer of data between hospitals, many

hospital staffs have extensive contacts with the outside world via their modems (Janczewski/Singh, 1999).

As a result of the above tendencies, hospitals are turning their interest mainly to monitor access to their IS. But as soon as the access is granted, a few more restrictions apply. Taking into account the existing modem connections, one may conclude that in general terms hospital information systems are quite vulnerable to attacks both from outside and inside.

One of the ways of reducing probability of an attack is to increase

Fig 5: Reference Monitor Architecture

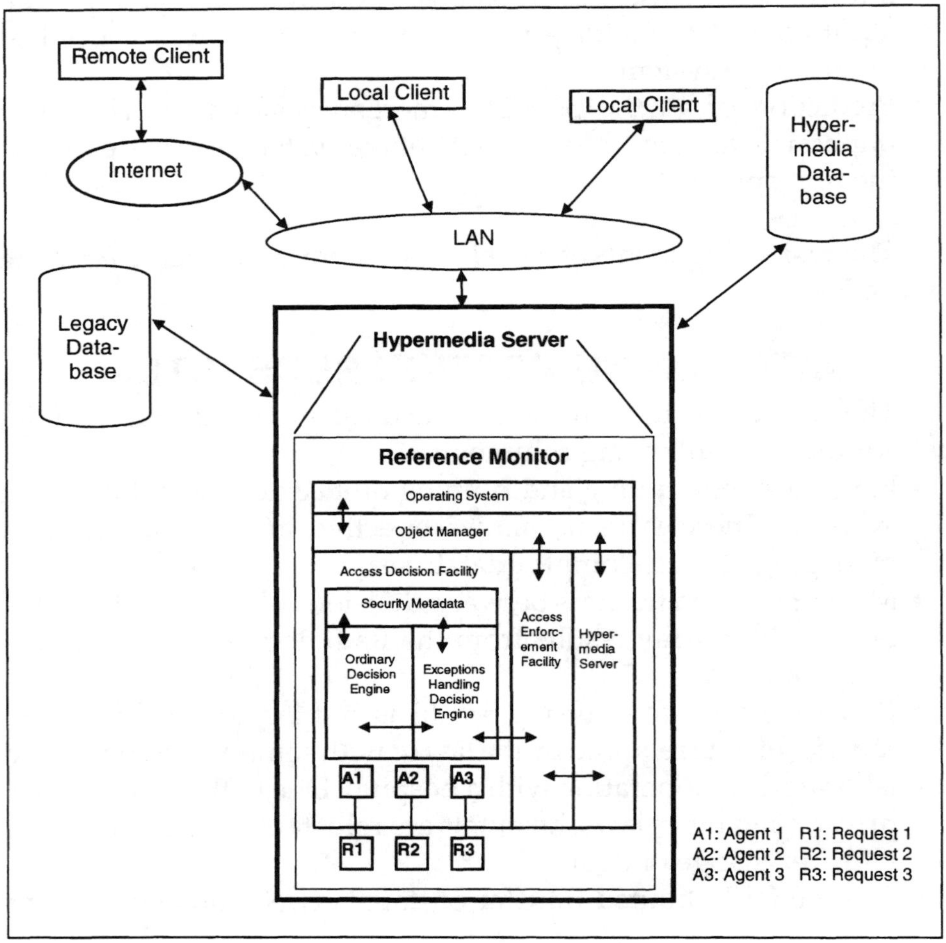

security of the telecommunication part of the medical information systems. In doing so, several rules should be followed.

With the exception of the basic personal information, there is not need to encrypt the majority of transmitted data as long as the record ID would not be directly related to a patient. This means that, for instance, a batch of data from a blood analysis lab could be sent as plain text as long as the records of individual tests are not associated with patients but with one-off identifiers. On the other hand it is important to have a high degree of certainty that the records were indeed generated by the nominated party and were not changed during the transmission. This can be easily accomplished using asymmetric encryption and digital signatures. Such procedure could result in a package of data having a form presented in Figure 6.

The structure suggested in Figure 6 allows very quick assembly and is not expensive to arrange. As mentioned before, the basic medical information is sent in as a plain text form and the patient name is hidden behind the temporary patient's ID. As long as the patient's ID is recognisable for both parties involved in the transmission the privacy of the patient is protected. This means that the parties, prior to the exchange of information, should agree on the method of identifying the patients. By producing the hash of the message and the sender address, the receiving party could be assured that the data were not changed during the transmission as well as there was no spoofing of the sender identity.

To verify the identity of the sender, the sender's certificate must be included in the message. The X.509 Public-Key Certificates could be easily adopted here. Structure of an X.509 certificate is depicted in

Figure 6: Structure of a Medical Record in Transmission

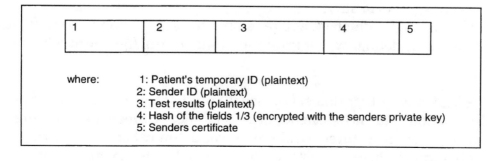

Figure 7: X.509 Public-Key Certificate

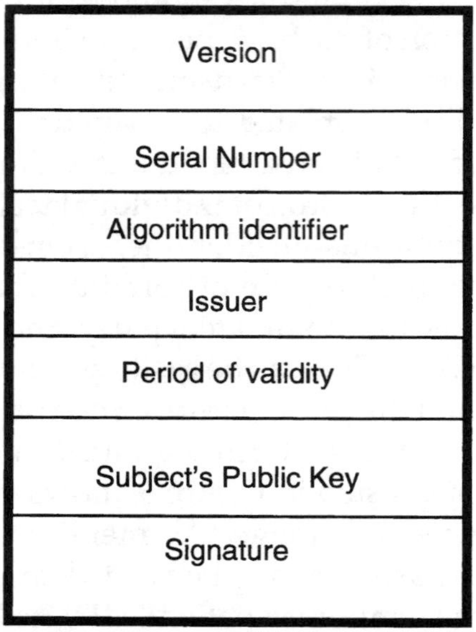

Version
Serial Number
Algorithm identifier
Issuer
Period of validity
Subject's Public Key
Signature

Figure 7.

All the above leads us to a conclusion that cryptographic protocols similar to the well-known Privacy Enhanced Mail (Schneier, 1993) using the simplest possible mode, MIC-CLEAR, would be sufficient to warrant proper secure transmission of medical records. It is assumed, however, that the parties involved in the transmission would agree on the method of generating and transmitting patient temporary IDs.

DATABASE SUBSYSTEM

The issue of security of databases, and medical databases in particular, could be examined from two perspectives:
- Security of a database as a by-product of a properly designed and managed IS facility.
- Security of a database as a resistance to actions aimed at destroying confidentiality, integrity and availability of the information in it.

This means that first set of issues could solve such problems as duplication, data inconsistency or dependence between the programs and the data structures, while the second could take care of more sophisticated threats. Castano, et al. (1995) lists several database protection requirements which are very appropriate for medical IS:

- **Protection from improper access**
  The basic access mechanism was covered in the section on reference monitor. Here it is important to mention problems of granularity, i.e., on what level the access would be located: whole database, records, attributes and values.

- **Protection from inference**
  In the medical databases many items are semantically related, thus allowing a user to come to know the value of a data item without accessing it directly, but inferring it from known values. By definition total protection against an inference attack is impossible to achieve, but there are methods of significantly reducing such a threat. One of the most popular is to refuse to present results of a query if the product of the query is based on three or less records.

- **Integrity of a database**
  This is a vast field covering protections from unauthorised access that could modify the contents of data, as well from errors, viruses, sabotages, or failures in the system that could damage stored data. This also includes the backup and recovery procedures.

- **Operational integrity of data**
  Simultaneous access of many users could introduce substantial disturbances to a database. One of the most recognised threats is the threat of locking the database. This could happen when two users simultaneously want to modify the same record. The concurrency manager is a mechanism that handles such threats.

- **Semantic integrity of data**
  In a database there must be a mechanism that will control data within prescribed boundaries. For instance, the blood bank could have blood records of only known types (like "O," "A," "B," etc.) or of a possible sugar content.

- **Accountability and auditing**
  One of the most important security features of a database is its audit trail where all the transactions are recorded. The audit trail would not stop damage of the data, but would keep a record of who, when, where, and what did. Knowledge of the existence of an audit trail is a good prevention mechanism. Also an audit trail can be used to help to restore the original content of a database.

- **Management and protection of sensitive data**
  Databases containing both public domain and sensitive data (medical records belong to this category) should have adequate protection mechanisms allowing the efficient utilisation of the database without compromising the security of sensitive information.
- **Confinement**
  Confinement is intended as the necessity to avoid undesirable information transfer between systems programs, for example transfer of critical data to unauthorised programs. Such transfers could be directed via authorised channels, memory channels or covert channels. Memory channel is a facility that allows data stored by one program to be read by another program. A covert channel is a communication facility that was not intended to be used by the authors/owners of the data.

Security mechanisms in databases include the following measures:
- Access control,
- Flow Control,
- Inference control.

Access control in medical databases could be divided into two categories. One is associated with an access to a "primary" database. A primary database is the collection of information being more or less uniform. For instance, it could be a database of a diagnostic laboratory containing results of all the blood tests. The other category, the "secondary" database, is a collection of pointers to all information associated with a given topic. It could be, for instance, a databank containing all information about a patient or all information about tuberculosis cases in the country.

The access control mechanism for a primary database is relatively simple as the rules of access could be easily set up and controlled. For instance, a person who is in charge of the lab and all the personnel involved in generating and maintaining the tests results should have access to relevant records. Some limits could be imposed such as that a person performing the blood tests should not have access to the part containing the urine test, etc. The access to the primary data should be managed at the level of organisation directly responsible to running the particular database. Taking for example the previously mentioned diagnostic lab, the access rules should be set up, run and controlled by the management of the lab.

As a result of running a secondary database, a user could request access to some particular data as well. It could be, for instance, a doctor in a hospital requesting the complete file on his/her patient, including the results of blood tests. In such cases a number of solutions is possible. One of them would be to provide access only if the request is concatenated with permission from a patient. Such a solution is highly restrictive and not always functional, especially in the case of emergencies. Others seem to be more practical: a request for access to particular data is granted if it is accompanied by the signature of an authorised organisation. For instance, Diagnostic Lab A would provide access to information on a particular patient if the request for access include an authorised signature of a Hospital H. That would require prior arrangement between these two institutions about the access rights to their information resources. As the result a request for access to a primary database from a secondary source could have a format as in Figure 8.

Upon receiving such request the addressee would find from the field "2" who is the sender, and with the help of fields 4 and 5 would confirm the identity of the sender. Then the addressee would check if the sender is on the list of authorised database user and eventually grant the access.

The other aspect of the database security is the control of information flow. Flow control is exercised when there is a check to determine

Figure 8: Structure of a Request for Medical Data

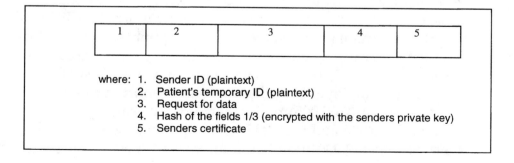

where: 1. Sender ID (plaintext)
        2. Patient's temporary ID (plaintext)
        3. Request for data
        4. Hash of the fields 1/3 (encrypted with the senders private key)
        5. Senders certificate

if a data flow from object X to Y does not violate all the security rules. For instance Object Y could have lower security clearance or on the way between X and Y, the data could be temporarily stored in less protected domain. Flow-control policies require admissible flows to be listed or regulated. Well-known security models like Bell-LaPadula or Biba are examples of flow-control policies.

Inference attacks happens when an unauthorised party attempts to gets data not through direct query (which could be declined) but through accessing another set of data and then deriving the required information. The classical example is an attempt to locate an HIV-positive patient in a small community. Assuming that HIV tests are carried with a frequency no higher than one person per day all that we need to know is who was referred for the HIV tests and how many more HIV positive patients are recorded for this community. Matching these two queries would easily yield the result, i.e., the name of the new HIV case in the community.

Books on database design (McFaddem, 1994) and security (Castano, 1995) abound with descriptions of methods decreasing the possibility of successful inference attack. As stated before, total protection against this type of attack is not possible, but many techniques exist which are able to reduce significantly the danger of such attacks.

The two most popular techniques are the following:

- **Data perturbation**
  Original items are replaced by microstatistic information, so the resulting global values are not changed but no single item is left in the database. For example, we cannot find how many square meters of space any given patient has, but we can have information about the average space per patient per ward.

- **Query size**
  This technique has already been mentioned. It is based on setting the limit on which a query set could be executed. For example, let us assume that we would try to find out how much the CEO of a hospital is earning (if this value is not in the public domain). We can start querying the database "How many people are earning per annum," in $5,000 increase steps. As CEO is usually the highest paid employee in an organisation a report that no person earns more than $100,005 implies that the CEO's earnings must be between $100,000 and $100,005, assuming that the result of the query on the $100,000 brought the answer "1". If we would set up

the limit on three records, then the query after $85,000 should stop reporting. That would leave us with information that there are at least three people in the company receiving more than $80,000, but we would not be able to pinpoint the CEO and his/her salary nor the other two staff.

CONCLUSIONS

In this chapter we presented the most important issues relating to the security of medical information systems.

Medical information systems have grown significantly in the last 10 years. From small ward-centred systems processing textual information, they have become systems storing and processing most of the medical data irrespective of its format. Also, the accessibility of the information is widening; the data could be reached from anywhere in the world.

The majority of governments have introduced laws protecting the privacy of people and patients in particular. This makes the medical systems unique: protection of data is not only the issue of well being of the organisation running the system, but also is subject to scrutiny of the law of a country. This means that the management of the medical information systems must take real care of the way they are running the medical IS.

The rapid growth of the Internet has added the next important factor to the issue of medical systems' security. With over 150 million users spread all over the world (estimates from June 1999), the probability of intentional or non-intentional system abuses is growing exponentially. Management must be aware of these threats and act accordingly with dire consequences of non-action.

In this chapter we presented a review of the most important issues related to the security of medical information systems. We would like to end this chapter by quoting two quite interesting aspects of the system security:

1. Two years ago the magazine *Fortune* (Behar, 1997) reported a case of a "tiger team" launching attacks on top companies from the Fortune 500 companies list. *Tiger team* is a nickname for a group of specialists who, with the knowledge of the top management, is trying to break into a corporate information system in an attempt to find the weak spots of the line of defence. In this particular case

the tiger team was not able to penetrate through the firewall software protecting the company computers. However, after several hours the team was able to obtain the status of the system administrator with total control of the whole company IS resources (including authority to change/delete of all the records!) through the unlisted modems hooked to the system. One can imagine the consequences of such an attack against a medical information system.

2. Attaining total security of information systems is not possible. However there is a simple 20/80 rule which says that with 20 percent of the budget, you could protect 80% of the resources. In other words, with a relatively low budget you could dramatically improve the security of your system.

REFERENCES

Amoroso, E. (1994). *Fundamentals of Computer Security Technology*, Prentice-Hall International, Englewood Cliffs, USA.

Behar, R. (1997). Who's reading your email?, *Fortune*, No 3, USA.

Castano, S. et al. (1995). *Database Security*, Addison-Wesley, Wokingham, UK.

Holbein, R. & Teufel,S. (1995).A Context Authentication Service for Role Based Access Control in Distributed Systems – CARDS, *Proceedings of the 11th Conference of IFIP TC11*, Chapman & Hall, London, UK.

Janczewski, L., Lo, B. (1998). Reference Monitor For Hypermedia-Based Hospital Information Systems, *Proceedings of the 14th International Conference of IFIP TC 11*, Wien, Austria.

Janczewski, L.J. Singh, P.P. (1999). Data Communication Security Issues for Multi-Media Hospital Information Systems, *Proceedings of the 1999 IRMA Conference*, Hershey, USA.

Keng, B.P. (1998). Privacy Protection in a Hypermedia Health Information Network, MCom Thesis, Department of MSIS, The University of Auckland, Auckland, New Zealand

Longworth, E. (1995). The Law on Data Security and Privacy, Notes for lectures for the University of Auckland, Department of MSIS, Auckland, New Zealand.

McFaddem F., Hoffer, J. (1994). *Modern Database Management*, The Benjamin/ Cummings Publishing, Redwood City, USA.

Nyanchama, M., Osborn, S. (1994). Access Rights Administration in Role-Based Security Systems in Database Security, *VIII Status and Prospects IFIP*, North Holland: Elsevier Science B.V., England.

OECD (1992). Information Computer Communications Policy, Guidelines For the Security of Information Systems, *OECD/GD* (92) 190, Paris, France

Pangalos,G., el al. (1995). Improving the Security of Medical Database Systems, *Proceedings of the 11th Conference of IFIP TC11*, Chapman & Hall, London, UK.

Privacy Commissioner (1993). *Health Information Privacy Code*, Government Printer Wellington, New Zealand.

Privacy Commissioner (1993). *Privacy Act 1993*, Government Printer, Wellington, New Zealand.

Privacy Commissioner (1998). *Necessary and Desirable, Privacy Act 1993 Review*, Office of the Privacy Commissioner, Wellington, New Zealand.

Schneier, B. (1995). *E-mail Security*, Wiley, New York, USA

Chapter IV

Health Information Management and Individual Privacy: Application of New Zealand's Privacy Legislation

Felix B. Tan and Gehan Gunasekara
The University of Auckland

The chapter reports on recent developments in the management of health information in New Zealand and the implications these initiatives have raised regarding individual privacy. Set up in 1993 to implement the country's health information strategy, the New Zealand Health Information Service (NZHIS) has recently established a national health register. At the heart of this development are three national databases: the National Health Index, the Medical Warnings System and the National Minimum Data Set. These applications and their functions are presented. Also discussed is a number of other health information management initiatives currently being explored.

The chapter contends that these initiatives under the guise of advancing the nation's health may, instead, be infringing the privacy and confidentiality of the nation's citizens. The chapter further considers the application of New Zealand's privacy legislation (the Privacy Act 1993 and the Health Information Privacy Code) to the development of centralised health information management systems. It concludes by considering the possibility of hidden agendas despite the provisions of the nation's privacy rules.

INTRODUCTION

Purchasing and providing health services is an information-intensive activity. Millions of pages of information are recorded every year. Much of the information is relevant to the ongoing care of individuals. However, health information is plagued with problems of access, duplication and interpretation. Health information management in New Zealand is no exception. For example, the nation's health professionals requiring information for the care and treatment of patients have had to rely on fragmented information flows—as information needed for care or treatment of patients is collected at various sources. As a result, these professionals find it difficult to obtain relevant information in a timely and cost effective manner. There is a consensus in the country's health sector that the existing systems and organisational arrangements do not meet current needs and will not easily accommodate the requirements of the health sector reforms and the information needs of the future. In response to this, the 1991 Health Information Strategy outlines a framework for the development of health information services to meet the national requirements for health information.

This chapter essentially describes recent developments in health information management in New Zealand initiated by the proposals in the 1991 Health Information Strategy. It discusses the role of the New Zealand Health Information Service (NZHIS) in the development of a national health register. It also considers the issue of privacy and confidentiality of the collection and use of health information. The chapter argues that there is more than meet the eye. The government purports that a centralised health information management system should result in better health delivery by freeing up health resources (Ministry of Health, 1996), but at whose expense?

To set the scene, the chapter begins with a background and an overview of the country's health information management. A review of the health information strategy initiative and a description of what has been implemented follows. A discussion of the issues around privacy and confidentiality ensues with special focus on the nation's privacy rules. It concludes by questioning the real motives of the New Zealand Health Sector and its Government for developing a centralised health register. The chapter suggests that to date the initiatives have failed to take into account and comply with New Zealand's stringent privacy rules.

HEALTH INFORMATION MANAGEMENT IN NEW ZEALAND

Up to and until the early 1990s, health information at a national level was provided and used by the then area health boards, private hospitals and the Department of Health (Ministry of Health, 1991). A review of the health information systems and related services then identified significant problems with the existing national collections and services. Some of these problems related to (i) lack of quality standards and standard data definitions; (ii) problems of data accessibility and timeliness; (iii) uncoordinated and overlapping points of collection; and (iv) a poorly maintained National Master Patient Index. The review concluded that the current systems do not meet existing needs, neither are they able to accommodate the new requirements of the future or the new requirements of the health sector reforms. A further conclusion was that new data systems, processing and organisational structures are necessary to support the development of world class healthcare provision and management. There was a considerable consensus between, and within, working groups involved in the review on the need for change and the direction of that change.

In 1991, a national health information strategy was developed as a collaborative effort by the country's health sector (Ministry of Health, 1991). The strategy was designed to address the lack of relevant, timely, and accurate information. It provided a national framework for the development of health information services to meet the national requirements for health information. The strategy suggested the need to establish a new entity—the National Health Information Service—to manage the national health information services in New Zealand. This new entity, described in the next section, would streamline many of the current activities and manage the services as a business.

NZ HEALTH INFORMATION SERVICE

The New Zealand Health Information Service (NZHIS) is a group within the Ministry of Health responsible for the collection and dissemination of health-related information. It was set up in 1993 to implement the country's health information strategy. Its primary goal is to make accurate information readily available and accessible in a timely manner throughout the health sector. The NZHIS therefore has responsibility for all aspects of health information management — from the collection, processing, maintenance and distribution of health data and statistics to the continuing development and maintenance of a national health information system, including the provision of appropriate databases, systems and information products (NZHIS, 1997a). The vision of NZHIS is to support the health sector's ongoing effort to improve health information management in New Zealand. The NZHIS recently established a national health register which may be the envy of many larger, wealthier countries (Sybase, 1998). This centralised repository of health information is summarised in the next section.

THE NATIONAL HEALTH REGISTER

The national health register consists of several core applications implemented on the Sun Microsystems platform with multi-CPU servers. Running over public electronic highways, these applications contain information for secondary and tertiary health events from Crown Health Enterprises (CHEs). At the heart of this development are three national databases: the National Health Index (NHI), the Medical Warnings System (MWS) and the National Minimum Data Set (NMDS). These have been designed to incorporate stringent safeguards to protect the information they hold from unauthorised access or misuse, but also to make crucial information about patients and their health available to authorised users for legitimate purposes.

National Health Index

The National Health Index (NHI) is a population-based register of all healthcare users (patients) in New Zealand. Assigned to each patient is a unique identifier allocated on a random basis. The NHI holds details such as names, alternate names, addresses, date of birth, gender and ethnicity. This enables an individual to be positively and uniquely identified for the purposes of healthcare services and records. The NHI number is in fact not a number but a string of seven characters, the first three of which are letters and the last four are numbers. Details of the core fields, which are recorded in the NHI database for an individual, can be perused at NZHIS's online publication (http://www.nzhis.govt.nz/publications/NHI-MWS.html).

The NHI is developed essentially to help protect personally identifiable health data, particularly data held on computer systems, and to enable linkage between different information systems while still protecting privacy. Access to the NHI is therefore restricted to authorised users and is permitted by the Health Information Privacy Code 1994, under the Privacy Act 1993 (NZHIS, 1997b).

Medical Warnings System

The Medical Warnings System (MWS) is designed to "warn" healthcare providers of the presence of any known risk factors that may be important in making clinical decisions about individual patient care (e.g., allergies, sensitivities, past significant history, etc). The MWS provides information on medical warnings and alerts, healthcare event summaries and donor information. These data are held nationally because of the clinical importance of quick access to the clinical information and the relative geographic mobility of the New Zealand population. This enables a provider anywhere in the country to obtain potentially life-saving information about a specific patient in their care, once the patient has been uniquely identified. The responsibility for making sure that the content of the MWS is up to date will rest primarily with its users, the healthcare providers (NZHIS, 1997b).

National Minimum Dataset

The National Minimum Dataset (NMDS) is a single integrated collection of health data required at a national level for policy formulation and performance monitoring and evaluation. The NMDS provides a reliable, validated and comprehensive but selected set of information on (i) the health status of the New Zealand population; (ii) the factors which influence health status; (iii) health resources and their utilisation; (iv) the outputs, outcomes and impact of health services for national policy making; and (iv) the performance of the health sector (NZHIS, 1997a).

The NHI, MWS and NMDS are central to effective national health information management. In addition to these, the NZHIS also maintains a national cancer registry and records mental health events

(NZHIS, 1997a). The NZ Cancer Register has operated since 1948 and is a population-based tumor register of all primary malignant disease. It is regarded as one of the oldest cancer register in the world (Sybase, 1998). The mental health system is a register for all psychiatric patients currently in hospitals together with all admissions and discharges since 1974.

OTHER HEALTH INFORMATION MANAGEMENT INITIATIVES

Plans are now in place to expand the existing information base to include primary care information (NZHIS, 1997a). Considerable progress in this direction has been achieved, and various sites in primary care are operating with information systems that break new ground and offer significant advantages to patients, providers and purchasers. The use of electronic data interchange — for example, sending and receiving laboratory test orders and results or exchanging patient details for admission and discharge — is growing fast. Many provider groups are now making regular use of such facilities, or have pilot programs under way to explore their benefits. It will not be long before many of these programmes coalesce into larger groups offering more services and therefore greater benefits to both doctors and their patients (NZHIS, 1997b).

Although the core function of the NZHIS is the management of health information for the Ministry of Health, it has also established a business centre, offering its services on the open commercial market. The NZHIS has the flexibility to leverage its expertise to tender and bid for outside projects to generate additional revenue. An example of such external projects is the recent implementation of a pharmaceutical data warehouse. Funded by two commercial enterprises and in coordination with another agency responsible for managing pharmaceutical expenditure policy, the NZHIS was contracted to establish and store a data warehouse for all pharmaceutical information from across New Zealand (Sybase, 1998).

Every healthcare provider in New Zealand records and exchanges health information, and this is increasingly done in electronic format. The National Health Index (NHI) plays an important role in this process by providing a unique identifier for the whole health sector, including primary care. A wider use of the NHI would greatly improve the exchange of information between healthcare providers and make possible the integration of patient information from various sources. This can be facilitated by a Health Intranet (NZHIS, 1998). Pilot projects are currently underway to develop a proof of concept. This will test the practical benefits of the Health Intranet. When fully implemented, this initiative will provide a secure means of communications nationwide, with access to all health information systems for all healthcare providers registered to use the intranet.

ISSUES OF PRIVACY AND CONFIDENTIALITY

Most health information is collected in a situation of confidence and trust for the purposes of care and treatment. Assurances as to confidentiality and protection of privacy are vital components of the relationship between patient and health professional and are necessary if the latter is to obtain accurate information from the former in order to make an accurate diagnosis. It is therefore not surprising that the modern privacy rules overlap substantially with a much older law of confidentiality and the medical ethics of the profession. The notions of dignity and autonomy which underlie New Zealand's privacy law also have much in common with the idea of informed consent which is central to current medical practice (Slane, 1998a). Against this backdrop it is strange that there has been to date very little public outcry over the development of a centralised health register in this country. This can be explained by two possible reasons. Firstly, there appears to be a lack of public awareness of the implications of these developments. According to a recent report prepared for the New Zealand Privacy Commissioner (Stevens, 1998), the issue of health information has bypassed public scrutiny. There are still many details to be addressed and debated. The lack of discussion involving all parties concerned has resulted in many doctors and even more patients being unaware of the type of patient details which are going to be collated and kept by health authorities. The same report goes as far as to suggest that there is something disquieting about the way health information is being managed in this country, with the health sector exhibiting a lack of openness about the various developments and plans in the collection of individual health information. As this program moves forward, it seems appropriate that more attention should be given to consultation with the public and debate within parliament. However this is more than a matter of good public relations: it is a legal requirement of New Zealand's privacy regime that individuals about whom information is collected are informed as to the purposes of the collection as well as the intended recipients of it.

Secondly, it might be thought that there is a high level of acceptance and trust amongst New Zealanders that the information collected will be used appropriately. For instance, information can be used to catch people defrauding the system by matching data from various agencies like inland revenue, accident compensation and social welfare. Data matching has been a practice since the middle of 1998. Television commercials advising the public about inter-agency data matching serve as a warning about defrauding the government. According to a senior health official interviewed by the author, the general population appears to be comfortable with the concept of a health number for tracking hospital admission and discharge; the use of a universal number by general practitioners; and the recording of allergies and health history on a national database. For example, Community Service Cards were first issued in the early 1990s, and today around 50% of the population carry them. These cards entitle cardholders to discounted consultations with general practitioners, but they do not contain the NHI number or any medical information. It appears that people are often surprised that these cards are not linked to their medical details and do not give their NHI number when swiped. An 'improvement' to this card is currently underway in the form of a medical smart card pilot. The smart cards combine Community Service Card details, NHI number and medical warnings of the cardholder. New Zealanders have a strong history in accepting the use of electronic systems, with the highest penetration of EFTPOS terminals in the world (New Zealand Bankers Association, 1995). This may explain the high level of acceptance of the development of a centralised health information system and the use of electronic health cards in this country.

On the other hand such acquiescence on the part of the general population cannot be assumed to exist. In the first place, while it is true that various data matching schemes between government departments exist (the Privacy Commissioner is empowered to sanction such schemes provided there are certain safeguards), the data matching schemes are targeted at what is perceived to be a minority antisocial element in the population. It is a very different thing to build up comprehensive health profiles of every single person, including law-abiding citizens. Furthermore reported complaints to the Privacy Commissioner provide evidence that ordinary citizens are particularly sensitive about their health information or about the potential misuse by health agencies of information about them.

In one case, for example, a customer complained when a pharmacy (where she was due to collect medicines which had earlier been out of stock) delivered medicines to her home without prior warning – it was a case of the extra customer service not being appreciated. While a simple phone call would have avoided the problem an interesting question arises as to whether delivering medicines are directly connected with the pharmacist's purpose for holding the customer's name and address. Another complaint arose over the wording of a form asking parents to consent to immunisation. The form did not state how the information would be used. It also contained a number without explanation. The complainant assumed that children had been allocated identification numbers and that the information would be entered into a database. In fact the number was simply a batch coding for the vaccines, so that if something went wrong with one of the batches, the affected children could be contacted. Apart from statistical data, the main use of the information was in fact to inform the children's doctors so they would know whether to offer immunisation. These cases show a keen awareness by members of the public of their right to privacy.

NEW ZEALAND'S PRIVACY REGIME

At first sight New Zealand has a privacy regime which is well geared to the challenges posed by the development of a national health register. The Privacy Act 1993 (the Act) is radical in its application as it applies to both the public and private sectors – it applies to all "agencies" which are defined so widely that even individuals are subject to the Act. The Act governs the collection, use and disclosure of "personal information" (information about identifiable individuals). The Act also entitles individuals to access information held about them. Most importantly, the Act is *information* based, not *document* based. It does not therefore matter whether the information is stored or transferred through electronic means or through paper files – the same rules apply.

Central to the Act are the 12 Information Privacy Principles (Slane, 1997). For instance Information Privacy Principle 1 (IPP 1) requires that only information necessary for a lawful purpose of the agency is collected and that the collection must be necessary for that purpose. However, this is also good information management practice. While the design of any data system proceeds backwards from the required outputs, one of the major health agencies recently put under scrutiny has been criticised because its outputs were evolving rather than having been stated at the outset (Stevens, 1998). IPP 3 is particularly important. It requires that an individual from whom information is collected is not only made aware of the fact of collection but also informed of the purposes for the collection and the intended recipients of the information. This most basic of requirements is evidently not always complied with, especially when frontline healthcare providers are required to forward information about patients to central funding authorities (Slane, 1998a).

IPP 3 is relevant to Information Privacy Principles 10 and 11. IPP 10 requires that information held about an individual only be used for the purpose for which it was collected or for a directly related purpose. IPP 11 requires that personal information held by an agency not be disclosed outside that agency unless such disclosure is one of the purposes in connection with which the information was obtained, or is a directly related purpose. A crucial point here is that the purpose of the collection must be at the time of collection of the information. In other words, the purpose must have been communicated to the data subject (IPP 3). Otherwise, an agency could arbitrarily make up purposes for the information as it went along, or think of new uses for information it already has. This is contrary to the requirements of the Act. If the information is to be used or disclosed for purposes different to those articulated at the outset, consent must be sought from the individuals concerned.

One of New Zealand's major funding authorities (North Health) has been at the forefront of moves towards integrating primary health information (doctors and pharmacies) into its data depository. Through use of the NHI number, the authority plans to collate and track individuals' attendance with different doctors, specialists, pharmacies, hospitals and other clinics over their entire lifetime (Stevens, 1998). However, in brochures encouraging the use of the NHI number, no explanation was offered as to the information which would be collected through its use or as to the ultimate uses and recipients of it. More seriously, in terms of IPP 3, no purposes for the compilation of the information were clearly stated. It has been rightly pointed out that while the agency may have been merely seeking to gather as much information as it could while not yet having formulated uses for it, such an approach is anathema to the Privacy Act (Stevens, 1998). The end of this discussion will focus on the real motives for establishing centralised health information management and as to whether any of these goals are sanctioned by the privacy regime.

Other Information Privacy Principles are of significance for centralised health information management. IPP 5 is the only principle specifically addressing the security of storage of information. The Privacy Commissioner has observed that the focus of the Act is not only in stopping leaks, but also in determining where the pipes lead (Slane, 1998b). IPP 8 requires that agencies take steps to ensure information is accurate prior to using it—a step that would seem especially relevant in the health context. IPP 9 requires that information be retained for no longer than necessary. Last but not least is IPP 12, which relates to unique identifiers. Among other things, IPP 12 prohibits an agency from assigning to an individual the same unique identifier that has been assigned by another agency. It will shortly be seen that this last requirement has been specifically modified in relation to use of the NHI number.

It should also be noted briefly that the information privacy principles are, for the most part, not enforceable through the courts but rather through an alternative dispute resolution procedure. This procedure begins with the Privacy Commissioner (who acts in the first place as a conciliator), although a complaint can be taken to a tribunal, which has considerable powers including the award of damages.

There are a number of qualifications and exceptions to the Information Privacy Principles. Some of these are stated within the principles themselves, for instance non-compliance for law enforcement and public health and safety purposes. Another common exception is where information is collected for research or statistical purposes, provided it is to be published in a non-identifiable form. There are also grounds for denying access to personal information under IPP 6.

The principles generally provide that non-compliance may be authorised by the individual concerned. This has the potential to cause serious mischief, particularly when agencies regard consent as a panacea. There is always the tendency to regard a one-off consent as sufficient. Consent must be not only informed but genuine. In the health arena patients are at the receiving end of an unequal power relationship and the Privacy Commissioner has referred to the "façade of patient control" (Slane, 1998b).

Finally the Privacy Commissioner is empowered to modify the information privacy principles (by prescribing greater or lesser standards than contained in the principles) in relation to specified matters by issuing codes of practice, which have the same force as the principles. This allows flexibility in adjusting the Act to the requirements of particular industries or types of information. Not surprisingly, one of the first codes of practice to be promulgated (there have so far been very few) was the Health Information Privacy Code 1994 (the Code) which is discussed next.

HEALTH INFORMATION PRIVACY CODE

In the introduction to the code, three special characteristics of the health sector and health information are cited as the rationale for a separate code. These are: firstly, confidentiality of collection (in the context of a confidential relationship); secondly, the nature of the information (highly sensitive); and thirdly, ongoing use (health information may be required long after it has ceased to be needed for the original episode of care and treatment). It will be observed that of these the first two at least provide justification for more stringent standards than in the Act.

Despite this, the Code itself is an unremarkable document. The 12 Health Information Privacy Rules broadly follow the Information Privacy Principles. Perhaps the most useful feature is a detailed commentary, which is no doubt useful to health professionals. There are some modifications of the privacy principles. From the point of view of the present discussion, the most significant alteration is in Rule 12(3) which allows specified agencies to assign the NHI number as an unique identifier. There are some safeguards. For instance, Rule 12(6) provides that an agency must not require an individual to disclose any unique identifier assigned to that individual unless the disclosure is for one of the purposes in connection with which that unique identifier was assigned or for a directly related purpose.

However as was observed earlier, it is extremely doubtful if these purposes have been communicated to the individuals concerned or indeed even articulated in the first place.

Rule 12(6) and its parent IPP 12(4) are seriously flawed for another reason. They do not preclude the unique identifier being obtained from someone other than the individual concerned. In the moves described earlier by the funding authorities towards building up a data depository one of the steps has been to require every claim for subsidy payments (most prescriptions and laboratory tests as well as some doctors visits are subsidised by the government in New Zealand) to be accompanied by the NHI number of the patient concerned. It is easy to see how an otherwise reluctant profession can be coerced into supplying the number. Yet as currently worded, they can be made to disclose the number for any purpose whatever.

The lack of adequate safeguards here is disappointing. When New Zealand's first privacy legislation was enacted in 1991, it served as a convenient smokescreen to allow the government to proceed with plans for data matching. There is a danger that the code will encourage similar complacency. Indeed it appears that the Health Ministry's statement in its Web site that the Privacy Commissioner was involved in ensuring the highest standards of privacy were without foundation – the office had not even been consulted (Stevens, 1998).

HIDDEN AGENDAS?

What are the possible motives or the rationale for centralised health information management? A number of possible explanations have been given (Stevens, 1998). No doubt the fundamental concern (in New Zealand as in other developed nations) has been to control the cost of healthcare to the government. One suggestion has been for "capitation" systems where individual customers are enrolled with a health management organisation and identified each time they seek a healthcare service so that costs can be referred back to the responsible organisation. If information is power then an interesting application of a complete patient database is a means of wresting power away from the doctors who are seen as currently accountable to nobody for their economic efficiency.

Another explanation has been that the new systems will eliminate or reduce the incidence of fraud (especially over state healthcare subsidy payments). However these claims (for instance that as much as 11% of all claims are fraudulent) have been ridiculed – if hundreds of millions of dollars were indeed being lost, it is hard to explain why to date little or no efforts have been spent on audit and fraud detection. In any case it is extremely doubtful that the elimination of waste is covered by the ambit of the law enforcement exceptions to the privacy principles.

A more radical plan has been hinted at. This is to set up, for planning purposes, a database which records, for every individual in New Zealand, a substantial degree of detail about symptoms as well as diagnoses and treatments (using a set of standard codes), and captures every healthcare transaction and the cost of that transaction whether or not it is state funded. Such a database would be a world first, and may well set New Zealand up as the world's foremost health research field and testbed. However, such lofty goals (even if they exist) have not been articulated at the level of the individuals concerned which, as explained earlier, is a clear violation of New Zealand's privacy regime.

Cogent reasons exist, on the other hand, for not relying on centralised medical records. In making diagnosis and treatment decisions, good medical practice suggests not trusting information recorded by others, especially where the accuracy of the information is vital. There is little or no empirical research linking better patient health outcomes with centralised medical records. Hence, a full and accessible patient health record may not necessarily be beneficial to the patient.

Finally, the authors argue that a less benevolent possibility exists for the use for centralised health records. If the tentative steps taken so far in New Zealand eventually mature into a comprehensive centralised record for every individual then it will be possible to give every individual a classification as either a good, average or bad health "risk." The utility of such information to insurance companies is obvious. It has been fashionable for some time, in New Zealand, to take an "insurer" view of health spending. There have been proposals for privatisation and accompanying cuts in government health spending. One possibility, which may be attractive to the government, will be the "farming out" of certain patients to the private sector. The existence of a precise "risk assessment" mechanism will undoubtedly assist this process.

CONCLUSION

In summary, this article briefly outlines recent developments in health information management in New Zealand. A centralised national health register is now in place with a few thousand PCs linked to a central IT client/server platform. This system now services around 30 hospitals and other medical services providing health care to New Zealand's 3.6 million population. The resolution of a number of issues pertaining to individual privacy and medical ethics are the current challenges facing the nation.

While New Zealand possesses a highly developed body of privacy rules which clearly apply to the initiatives highlighted, these are evidently not always complied with. The privacy rules mandate the fostering of greater public awareness of the uses of information. To date this has been lacking. It remains to be seen how effective the Privacy Commissioner will be in his potentially powerful role in monitoring and regulating the initiatives for centralised health information management.

REFERENCES

Ministry of Health (1991). *Health information strategy for New Zealand, 1991.*

Ministry of Health (1996). *Improving our health information system.* Http://www.health.govt.nz/HIS2000/general/his2000_news.html.

New Zealand Bankers Association (1995) *Annual review 1995,* Wellington.

NZHIS (1997a). *Data & services.* Http://www.nzhis.govt.nz/Service_guide.html.

NZHIS (1997b). *National Health Index and Medical Warning System.* Http://www.nzhis.govt.nz/publications/NHI-MWS.html.

NZHIS (1998) *Health intranet project.* Http://www.nzhis.govt.nz/projects/intranet.html.

Slane, B. (1997). *Information privacy principles.* Http://www.privacy.org.nz/people/fact3-0.htm.

Slane, B. (1998a). *Centralised databases: People, privacy and planning.* A paper presented by the Privacy Commissioner to the New Zealand - Australia Health IT Directors Meeting, 18 February.

Slane, B. (1998b). *Information protection in healthcare: Knowledge at what price?* Address by the Privacy Commissioner to the Health Summit '98, 15 July.

Stevens, R. (1998). *Medical record databases: Just what you need?* A Report for the Privacy Commissioner, April.

Sybase (1998). *NZHIS health register*, Sybase, 1st Quarter, 16-17.

Chapter V

Understanding Success and Failure of Health Care Information Systems

Richard Heeks, David Mundy and Angel Salazar
University of Manchester, UK

INTRODUCTION

Some health care information systems (HCIS) do succeed, but the majority are likely to fail in some way. To explain why this happens, and how failure rates may be reduced, the chapter describes the "ITPOSMO" model of conception-reality gaps. This argues that the greater the change gap between current realities and the design conceptions (i.e., requirements and assumptions) of a new healthcare information system, the greater the risk of failure.

Three archetypal large design-reality gaps affect the HCIS domain and are associated with an increased risk of failure:

- *Rationality—reality gaps*: that arise from the formal, rational way in which many HCIS are conceived, which mismatches the behavioral realities of some healthcare organizations.
- *Private—public sector gaps*: that arise from application in public sector contexts of HCIS developed for the private sector.
- *Country gaps*: that arise from application in one country of HCIS developed in a different country.

Some generic conclusions can be drawn about successful approaches to HCIS development. Examples include the need for more reality-oriented techniques and applications, and greater use of participative approaches to HCIS. More specifically, techniques can be identified for each of the seven ITPOSMO dimensions that will help close the gap between conception and reality. This can include the freezing of one or more dimensions of change. Such techniques will help improve the contribution that information systems can make in healthcare organizations.

Overall, then, this chapter will provide readers with an understanding and model of why healthcare information systems succeed or fail, and with general guidance on how to avoid HCIS failure.

BACKGROUND: HEALTH CARE INFORMATION SYSTEM SUCCESS AND FAILURE

New information systems have a powerful potential to improve the functioning of healthcare organizations (Neumann et al., 1996; Raghupathi, 1997). However, that potential can only be realized if healthcare information systems can be successfully developed and implemented.

There are a large number of reported HCIS success stories from around the world, but these seem likely to be painting a falsely positive picture. There is generic evidence that a significant majority of information systems initiatives are failures in both the private sector (Korac-Boisvert and Kouzmin, 1995; James, 1997) and the public sector (Heeks and Davies, 1999).

There is also plenty of specific evidence that many – even most – healthcare information systems are failures. Anderson's (1997:90) work on HCIS cites "studies that indicate half of all computer-based information systems fail." Keen (1994a:1) notes that, "For every documented success, there seems to be a clutch of failures." Likewise, Paré and Elam (1998:331) state: "Research shows that many healthcare institutions have consumed huge amounts of money and frustrated countless people in wasted efforts to implement information systems."

The same message of failure is also found in studies of particular healthcare applications. Many electronic patient record initiatives have failed (Dodd and Fortune, 1995) so that systems in the U.S. "still consist largely of paper records" (Anderson, 1997:89). So, too, for hospital information systems (HIS): "It appears that the set of all successful HIS implementations is only slightly larger than the null set, and these have usually been developed at academic center." (Rosenal et al., 1995:554).

In all, we can identify four main forms of HCIS failure:

- The *total failure* of a system never implemented or in which a new system is implemented but immediately abandoned. A much-reported example is that of the London Ambulance Service's new computerized dispatching system. This suffered a catastrophic failure within hours of implementation, leaving paramedics unable to attend healthcare emergency victims in a timely manner (Health Committee, 1995).

- The *partial failure* of an initiative in which major goals are unattained or in which there are significant undesirable outcomes. Anderson (1997:87), for instance, cites the case of "An information system installed at the University of Virginia Medical Center [*which*] was implemented three years behind schedule at a cost that was three times the original estimate."

- The *sustainability failure* of an initiative that succeeds initially but then fails after a year or so. Some of the case mix systems installed under the UK National Health Service's Resource Management Initiative fall into this category. They were made fully operational and achieved some partial use but with limited enthusiasm from staff for using them. Ultimately, they were just switched off (HSMU, 1996).

- The *replication failure* of an initiative that succeeds in its pilot location but cannot be repeated elsewhere. Although presenters may not realize it at the time, every health informatics conference is jam-packed with replication failures about to happen; with wonderful innovations that are tested once and then disappear without trace. As an audience, we hear all about the pilot, but we tend not to hear about the replication failure.

This all points to a yawning gap between the positive potential for information systems to contribute to the work of healthcare organizations and the largely negative reality. This, in turn, means that increasingly large sums of money are being invested in new health care information systems but that a substantial proportion of this will go to waste on unimplemented or ineffective systems.

Clearly, something must be done to try to reduce this wastage. To do this, we need to understand why failures occur and why, less frequently, there are successes.

Understanding HCIS Success and Failure

Paré and Elam (1998:332) note that most past investigation into failure of HCIS has tended to be normative, focusing on "a set of managerial prescriptions which, taken as a whole, constitute the "ideal" way to implement an information system. Yet, despite these normative principles, many organizations and healthcare institutions find their attempts to make use of computer-based information systems fraught with difficulty."

In seeking to understand HCIS failure, we must therefore take an alternative route forward rather than the standard prescriptive "cookbook" approach. The starting point will be that of *contingency* that sees no single blueprint for success and failure in organizational change (Poulymenakou and Holmes, 1996; Paré and Elam, 1998). Instead, it must be recognized that there are situation-specific factors for each HCIS which will determine success and failure and, hence, strategies for success.

Inherent within most ideas of contingency is the idea of *adaptation*: of states of mismatch and match between and within factors and of the need to change in order to adapt systems so that there is more match than mismatch. In the context of overall organizational change, this is mainly described in terms of the need for adaptation of organizational structure to the organizational environment (Butler, 1991). In the context of HCIS, too, there is an "environment" to which the information system can be adapted.

We will investigate this in greater detail in the following section but will note two key points here. First, that we are not just talking about matching the technological environment:

"Past experience suggests that efforts to introduce clinical information systems into practice settings will result in failures and unanticipated consequences if their technical aspects are emphasized and their social and organizational factors are overlooked. ... Several decades of experience with computer-based information systems make it clear the critical issues in the implementation of these systems are social and organizational, not solely technical" (Anderson 1997:89).

Second, that these "social and organizational factors" are not just a question of relatively objective realities, such as work processes or organizational structures, but also of relatively subjective perceptions. Dodd and Fortune (1995) and Dhillon (1998), for example, note the role of stakeholder assumptions, expectations, and viewpoints in contributing to the failure of healthcare information systems. In particular, these authors and Roberts and Garnett (1998) note that problems arise when there is a difference (i.e., a mismatch) between the model assumed within construction of the HCIS and the perceptions of key stakeholder groups such as medical practitioners.

Thus far, we can therefore conclude that a successful HCIS will be one that tends to match its environment in relation to technical, social and organizational factors; these latter including the perceptions of key stakeholders.

However, there is a major problem here: if the HCIS were to exactly match its environment, it would not change that environment in any way. Yet the formal purpose of HCIS is to support and bring about organizational change in order to improve the functioning of healthcare organizations. There must therefore be some degree of change that an HCIS introduces. Indeed, a greater degree of change may bring greater organizational improvements (though there is no necessary link between size of change and size of benefits).

On the other hand, if HCIS try to change too much this brings with it a risk of failure and, the more you change, the greater this risk (Dodd and Fortune, 1995). In the London Ambulance case, for example, failure arose because "the speed and depth of change were simply too aggressive for the circumstances" (Page et al., 1993, cited in Beynon-Davies, 1995:181). Equally, success becomes more likely when change is limited. For example, a successful patient record system in a UK hospital was implemented with a design that deliberately minimized cultural, work process, information and financial change (Roberts and Garnett, 1998).

Overall, then, there is a trade-off between change and risk for HCIS. Reducing the size of change may increase the chance of system success but also reduce the organizational benefits of that system. Conversely, increasing the size of change may reduce the chance of system success but also increase the organizational benefits of that system.

DIMENSIONS OF CHANGE: CONCEPTION — REALITY GAPS

From the previous section, we saw that central to healthcare information system success and failure is the amount of change between "where we are now" and "where the HCIS wants to get us."

The former will be represented by the current realities of the particular healthcare context (part of which may encompass subjective perceptions of reality). The latter will be represented by the model or conceptions and assumptions that have been incorporated into the new HCIS design. Putting this a little more precisely, then, we can say that success and failure depend on the size of gap that exists between "current realities" and '"design conceptions of the HCI."

Where do these design conceptions come from? They derive largely from the world view of those stakeholders who dominate the HCIS design process. We will discuss these in more detail later, but can note here that dominant stakeholders are typically drawn from technical or managerial or clinical groups. In this case, we should amend our earlier phrase from "where the HCIS wants to get us' to 'where the dominant stakeholders want the HCIS to get them."

Dimensions of the Conception-Reality Gap

Using a couple of HCIS case studies, we will now map out the dimensions of this "conception-reality gap."

Case Study 1

A "ComputerLink" scheme for 26 home-based AIDS patients was set up that put them in touch with each other individually and in groups, and with an encyclopedia (Brennan and Ripich, 1994). The scheme was a qualitative success, as judged by participant ratings, and a quantitative success, as judged by the fact that:
- ComputerLink was used, on average, 300 times during the six-month evaluation period by each patient;
- its private e-mail and public e-mail forum components were used more than 10,000 times; and
- its electronic encyclopedia of AIDS-related information was accessed nearly 800 times.

Its success can be attributed to the limited gaps that existed between the system's design conceptions (drawn largely from nurse and patient stakeholders) and contextual realities for the AIDS patients along seven dimensions:

- *An information dimension.* ComputerLink was designed in a way that offered great flexibility of information access either via the encyclopedia or via queries in public/private e-mail messages. Because of this conceptual flexibility, users were easily able to meet their real information needs through the system.

- *A technology dimension.* ComputerLink was designed around simple and straightforward technology using basic PCs, simple software and existing networking links. This therefore demanded relatively limited change along the technology dimension.

- *A process dimension.* ComputerLink was designed so that it supported the preexisting information-seeking and communication processes that AIDS patients undertook prior to computerization. There was thus virtually no gap between conception and reality along the process dimension.

- *An objectives and values dimension.* ComputerLink's design met patients' real needs and provided something they said was valuable to them: the ability to interact with other AIDS patients and to have more information about their condition. It was also designed to meet very different individual objectives, from those who wanted to interact with a group on a daily basis to those who wanted occasional individual communication or anonymous 'support' (from the encyclopedia).

- *A staffing and skills dimension.* ComputerLink was designed to require the input of only one project nurse on an irregular basis and to require only a limited number of new skills for system use. There was thus little gap between conceived and actual human capability requirements.

- *A management and structures dimension.* ComputerLink was designed to fit within the existing health structures and, as noted, required only the addition of a fairly simple management framework of one nurse to monitor the system.

- *An "other resources" dimension.* ComputerLink was designed to have very low implementation and operation costs, with equipment costing only US$350 per patient. Its financial requirements were therefore well matched to the real finances available. It was also designed to meet the time resource realities of patients by providing 24-hour access. Participants were therefore able to match expenditure of time to their availability periods. For example, there were as many logins between 10pm and 3am as between 10am and 3pm.

To sum up, the assumptions or conceptions underlying ComputerLink's design were either matched to existing realities or required only very limited change along seven possible dimensions. It was therefore successful because of its limited conception—reality gaps.

We can use this example to create a model of HCIS conception—reality gaps, which we will call the 'ITPOSMO' model because of its seven dimensions:

- **I**nformation
- **T**echnology
- **P**rocesses
- **O**bjectives and values
- **S**taffing and skills
- **M**anagement and structures
- **O**ther resources: money and time

Analysis of other information systems cases from both the healthcare sector (see below) and beyond (Heeks and Bhatnagar, 1999) indicates that these seven dimensions are necessary and sufficient to provide an understanding of conception—reality gaps.

Case Study 2

We can use the ITPOSMO model to explain HCIS failure as well as success. A UK hospital attempted to introduce an expert system for computerized coloscopy (Guah, 1998). However, the system design was conceived mainly by technical staff, and there were significant conception-reality gaps along a number of the ITPOSMO dimensions:

- *Information*: The expert system was designed to produce a set of statistical information on coloscopy, but it emerged that there was no significant demand for this information. There was thus a large gap between the information conceptions underlying the system and the information realities of existing hospital practice.
- *Technology*: The expert system required a relatively powerful

technological infrastructure, which differed markedly from the hospital's current technological realities.

- *Processes*: The expert system was designed to automate many of the currently human decision-making processes around coloscopy. This created a significant gap between the new processes conceived within the system design and the current process reality.
- *Objectives and values*: Because of the process automation, the system's design did not match well with the objectives and values of medical staff who feared automation and who believed that human inputs remained critical. Nor did the expert system's objectives match well with the priorities of senior hospital managers, leading to their providing little, if any, support for the project.
- *Staffing and skills*: the expert system was relatively difficult to use and there was thus a significant gap between the requirements of its design conceptions and the reality of availability and expertise of hospital staff.
- *Management and structures*: There was little conception—reality gap along this dimension.
- *Other resources*: The expert system was both time-consuming and costly to operate. This created a serious gap between the system's design requirements and the realities of resource availability within the hospital.

Overall, there was too great a gap between the design conceptions of the expert system and the realities of the hospital context into which it was being introduced. The result was that the pilot project was abandoned, having failed because of its outsize conception-reality gap.

ARCHETYPES OF HEALTH CARE INFORMATION SYSTEM FAILURE

Conception-reality gaps can arise in any situation, but we will highlight some archetypes that can make HCIS failure more likely.

Gaps Between Formal Rationality and Behavioral Reality

"Hard" rational models assume logic, formality and objectivity to underlie the workings of organizations. Alternative "soft" behavioral models of organizations have subsequently been developed. They assume factors such as human limitations, social objectives and subjectivity underlie the workings of organizations.

Difficulties occur in HCIS implementation where a hard rational design meets a soft behavioral reality. The design component can arise in a number of ways depending on which stakeholder group's world view dominates the HCIS design. Three archetypal examples will be provided here:

- *Technical rationality.* Technology is typically conceived as an objective and rational entity, not as something that incorporates particular cultural and political values. When information technology (IT) is seen to play a central role in HCIS, those information systems are therefore themselves likely to be conceived according to an objective and rational model. This may occur particularly, though not exclusively, where IT professionals dominate the design process, allowing a technology-based world view to dominate design conceptions. Isaacs (1995), Coiera (1997) and Dhillon (1998) report the tendency of IT personnel in healthcare to hold a rational, technology-focused world view:

  "Since the nature of IT exploitation within organizations is based on formal-rational models, analysts tend to study only the defined and official roles specified through job descriptions, etc. They do not consider the informal social relations, for example through coalition formulation, which are common in complex organizations" (Dhillon, 1998:10).

- *Managerial rationality.* Managers have their own objectives, but are also the conduit for the objectives of external stakeholder groups such as shareholders or governments. Such objectives can relate to legal or bureaucratic rationalities, but they frequently relate to money. Like technology, money is typically conceived as an objective and rational entity. When financial information is seen to play a central role in HCIS, those information systems are therefore themselves likely to be conceived according to an objective and rational model. This may occur particularly, though not exclusively, where healthcare managers dominate the design process, allowing a finance-based world view to dominate design conceptions. Both Ennals, et al. (1996) and Dhillon (1998) report the increasing imposition of rational financial management models via information systems as part of the healthcare reform process.

- *Medical rationality.* Although it deals with people, medicine is also frequently conceived in an objective and rational manner where diseases and injuries, not patients, are the focal entity (Keen, 1994a). When medical information is seen to play a central role in HCIS, those information systems are therefore themselves likely to be conceived according to an objective and rational model. This may occur particularly, though not exclusively, where doctors dominate the design process, allowing a medicine-based world view to dominate design conceptions.

The technical or managerial or medical world view incorporated into the HCIS' design conceptions may come into conflict with the actual and perceived realities of other healthcare stakeholders, especially practitioners, or it may not. Where it does conflict, there will be a large gap between the HCIS' formal, rational design conceptions and the more informal, behavioral realities of healthcare practitioners.

When there is such a gap, these behavioral realities should not simply be labeled "irrational" since they may derive from logically consistent viewpoints such as:

- *care rationality*: a viewpoint that sees the patient's needs as paramount; or
- *personal/political rationality*: a viewpoint that sees the stakeholder's own needs (or those of his/her group) as paramount.

Behavioral realities may equally derive from individual differences, human cognitive or other limitations, and from further viewpoints (including those which others would label "irrational").

It should be noted that gaps between formal, rational design and informal, behavioral reality are not always a case of disagreement between different stakeholder groups. They can also confuse individuals, making it difficult for them to "get in touch with reality"; for example, when trying to distinguish the information they think they ought to need from the information they actually need. Westrup (1998:84) similarly reports the difficulty health practitioners have in detaching themselves from dominant rational paradigms and recognizing what goes on in reality when describing processes:

"Nurses had problems in differentiating between what they actually did and what they said they did. So, for example, it is recognised that nursing as a profession should plan nursing care using a process of care planning. This is what nurses in the hospital I studied said they did and made a requirement of the [*new information*] system. In practice, care planning was seen as time-consuming and unnecessary for most nursing care ... As a consequence care planning was not done in practice. When the nursing system was implemented, care planning ... was embodied in the system and nurses had to create care plans if the system was to work properly. The upshot was that the computerised system was more time-consuming than previous practice."

Impacts of Imposing Rational Information Systems

Taking a patient perspective, we can classify three main impacts of imposing rational information systems on behavioral realities:

Potential benefits. There may be benefits in imposing more rational information systems on healthcare staff, where this suppresses behaviors based on selfish motives or on negative idiosyncrasies and human limitations. For example, research shows that 20-50% of major therapeutic intervention decisions, and perhaps a higher proportion of minor interventions, involve little or no use of the evidence base. As a result "proven useless and even frankly harmful therapies linger in practice long after the evidence is clear" (Davies and Nutley, 1999:12). Hence, there is a demonstrable need for – and value of – use of more rigorous and medically rational evidence-based information about the efficacy of health care interventions by healthcare practitioners.

Health care practitioners tend to resist change in this context because of a concern with preserving "long-standing practice patterns" (Anderson, 1997:84) and "their professional autonomy" (Beynon-Davies, 1995:181). We can view these as rather defensive reactions to the conception-reality gap.

Damaging impacts. There may be dangers in imposing more rational information systems on healthcare staff, where this suppresses patient-centered behaviors. For example, imposing rational information systems (IS) can suppress two important types of informal patient-centered information system. First are those that operate between health care professionals as an essential part of patient care (Davies, 1997). Second are those that operate between practitioners and patients, again as an essential part of patient care. As an example, problems often emerge when technically rational computerized knowledge-based systems are introduced into the patient consultation and diagnosis process (Steimann, 1995). The rational bias of one such system was evaluated:

"This was found to have at least two implications: the patient did not get the opportunity to air his [sic] own feelings and thoughts, and the dialogue switched back into past tense, focusing on the patient's problem history instead of the present situation." (Alendahl et al., 1995:919)

Healthcare practitioners tend to resist change in this context because of a concern about damaging healthcare outcomes (IMG, 1996; Greaves, 1998). From a patient perspective, we can view these as rather objectively-justifiable reactions to the conception-reality gap.

Equivocal impacts. As well as imposing rationality, rationally-conceived HCIS also tend to impose uniformity by allowing one particular way of doing things. This will suppress flexibility and diversity in the healthcare context, overriding the typical reality of individual work styles, needs and approaches (Lincoln and Essin, 1995). We term this an equivocal outcome since it may either help or hinder patient care. It may help in situations where flexibility and diversity are equated with corruption or with poor or uneven work quality. It may hinder in situations where flexibility and diversity are necessary reactions to individual patient and staff differences. Universal codes, for example, may improve the work of a poor medical practitioner but hinder the work of a good one (Ireland and Regan, 1995).

Outcomes of Imposing Rational Information Systems

A large gap between rational HCIS design conceptions and behavioral healthcare realities leads to the inevitable risks of failure.

Dhillon (1998), for example, reports the failure of a clinical information system in a UK hospital. The failure arose when the information system, based by its analysts on a formal, technically-rational model of hospital functioning, was introduced into a much "messier" informal reality, leading to "a clear mismatch between the formal models [*within the IS*] and the perceptions of system users who inevitably reflect a more informal and pragmatic approach to their own organizational realities" (Dhillon, 1998:2). There was a mismatch particularly along the process, objectives and structures dimensions of the ITPOSMO model. The "prescriptive and utterly inflexible" information system that resulted was of little use to health practitioners.

A patient assessment information system in the intensive care unit of a North American health center failed for similar reasons (Paré and Elam, 1998). It was designed according to a formal, managerially rational model of nursing that did not match realities. In particular, there was a conception-reality gap along the process and objectives dimensions of the ITPOSMO model:

- The computer system captured the time nurses made their system inputs and logged this as part of the legally submissible document that the system produced, since nurses "are requested by law to perform and document a complete assessment of each patient in the first 90 minutes of their shift." In reality, nurses sometimes found themselves needing to provide care to a critically ill patient immediately they came on shift. They were thus only able to document their assessments much later in the shift. It was easy to "work around" manual recording systems to incorporate this technically illegal but morally and clinically sound practice; but not so with the computerized system. Nurses adopted various means of coping with this conception-reality gap, including non-use of the computerized system.
- The computer system produced standardized reports. These demotivated the more experienced nurses who felt there was no way to demonstrate their additional value and expertise. The system's rational conception therefore failed to meet the reality of some nurse objectives and values, leading to their avoiding system use.

Gaps Between the Context of Design and of Implementation

As noted above, those who design healthcare information systems make certain assumptions that are then incorporated into the design. These assumptions will be at least partly determined by the context in which the HCIS was designed. For example, an HCIS designed in a context where preventive healthcare models are the norm may well incorporate certain preventive health model conceptions within it. This may not be problematic where the HCIS is then implemented within the same context in which it was designed. However, problems will arise if the design and implementation contexts are different.

We have already described *intra*-organizational examples of this in the previous section, where problems arose particularly due to the different contexts in which IT professionals, healthcare managers, and health care practitioners work. We can provide two further *inter*-organizational examples of this problem.

Public—Private Sector Gaps

We will focus the discussion here on hospitals, but the same issues arise for other public and private healthcare organizations.

Every hospital is different from every other hospital, creating a universal design-implementation context gap and, hence, problems —if one attempts to transfer an information system created in one hospital to another one (Gowing, 1994; McDaniel, et al., 1995). However, this gap is archetypally large between (depending on the national health system) public sector and private sector hospitals or nonprofit and for-profit hospitals. Differences exist between these two along all seven of the ITPOSMO dimensions. We will provide a few illustrative gaps here, based on Vogt, et al. (1996). These are stereotypes, and examples of reversals do exist, but they nonetheless represent typical gaps:

- *Information*: Public hospitals tend to place less emphasis on financial cost information and more emphasis on broader performance indicator information than private hospitals due to different regulatory requirements.
- *Technology*: Public hospitals tend to have a more limited and older technological infrastructure than that found in private hospitals.
- *Processes*: Public hospitals tend to treat a different case mix to private hospitals, typically treating far more illness of the poor, and thus requiring a rather different set of health intervention processes. Both administrative and clinical processes are also different because of the different funding arrangements for patients.
- *Objectives and values*: In the public sector, "such things as budget

maximization or output maximization have been posited as more plausible objectives ... By contrast, for-profit institutions hold profitability (and thus efficiency) as a primary goal" (Vogt et al., 1996:94).

- *Staffing and skills*: Public hospitals tend to have fewer nursing staff and fewer technology-related staff than private hospitals.
- *Management and structures*: public hospitals tend to have weaker non-clinical management and administration structures than private hospitals, partly due to different financing arrangements.
- *Other resources*: Public hospitals tend to have less money than private hospitals.

Given these differences, information systems or techniques developed for private sector hospital use can easily be based on conceptions that do not match public sector hospital realities. They will therefore be more prone to failure if introduced into a public sector hospital.

We will illustrate this not with a specific information system, but with a particular information systems technique: strategic information systems planning (SISP). SISP was designed within and for the private sector, and is based on conceptions of unitary organizational objectives, apolitical decision making, and the presence of skilled support for implementation that does not apply in many public sector healthcare organizations (Ballantine and Cunningham, 1999). This conception-reality mismatch has made traditional SISP risky and/or impractical in the public sector. This was epitomized in the UK public sector by cancellation of the Wessex Regional Health Authority's Regional Information Systems Plan, causing an estimated £20 million (c.US$33m) to be wasted (Beynon-Davies, 1995).

Country Gaps

Healthcare information systems developed in the context of one particular country will incorporate common assumptions of that context, but:

"Apart from the existence of a patient, a disease, and a doctor, one can sometimes question what is really common among the different health services and social welfare public systems existing throughout the world." (Dusserre et al., 1995:1476)

Every country is therefore different from every other country, creating a universal design-implementation context gap and, hence, problems — if one attempts to transfer an information system created in one country to another country. These gaps and HCIS transfer problems certainly exist between Western nations (Keen, 1994b; Curry, 1998). However, this gap and transfer problems are archetypally large between developing and industrialized countries (Vian, et al., 1993). Differences exist between these two along all seven of the ITPOSMO dimensions. We will provide a few illustrative gaps here, based on Heeks and Bhatnagar (1999):

- *Information*: Formal, quantitative information stored outside the human mind is valued less in developing countries.
- *Technology*: The technological infrastructure (telecommunications, networks, electricity, etc.) is more limited and/or older in developing countries.
- *Processes*: Work processes are more contingent in developing countries because of the more politicized and inconstant environment.
- *Objectives and values*: Developing countries are reportedly more likely to have cultures that value kin loyalty, authority, holism, secrecy, and risk aversion.
- *Staffing and skills*: Developing countries have a more limited local skills base in a wide range of skills. This includes IS skills of systems analysis and design, implementation skills, and operation-related skills including computer literacy and familiarity with the Western languages that dominate healthcare computing. It also includes a set of broader skills covering the planning, implementation and management of HCIS initiatives, and health care management.
- *Management and structures*: Developing country health care organizations tend to be more hierarchical and more centralized.
- *Other resources*: Developing countries have less money. In addition, the cost of IT is higher than in industrialized countries, whereas the cost of labor is less.

Perhaps even more than with the public-private gaps, it is important to recognize these as stereotypes and to remember that the Third World is not some computer-free wasteland. Countries like Iran, India and Morocco first introduced computers in the mid-1950s; computers are used today in many developing country hospitals; and some countries produce their own healthcare information systems. Vast gulfs also exist within industrialized countries: compare healthcare in Beverly Hills with that provided in South Central in Los Angeles, for instance.

Nonetheless, there is a major problem with the "If it works for us, it'll work for you" mentality being peddled round the Third World by IT and health care multinationals, by international consultants, and by aid donor agencies. Given the differences described, HCIS designed for use in an industrialized country can easily be based on conceptions that do not match realities in a developing country. They will therefore be more prone to failure if introduced into that developing country.

In the Philippines, an aid-funded project to introduce a field health information system was conceived according to a Western model that assumed the presence of skilled programmers, skilled project managers, a sound technological infrastructure, and a need for information outputs like those used in an American healthcare organization (Jayasuriya, 1995). In reality, none of these was present in the Philippine context, and the information system failed. Jayasuriya (1995:1604) concludes:

> "The alignment of IT to the organizational systems in developing countries tends to suffer from the assumption that models developed for developed countries are appropriate: this does not recognize the idiosyncracies of these systems."

Combining the Gaps

Where both sectoral and country gaps are combined, as occurred during the U.K.'s Resource Management Initiative, trouble is almost guaranteed. Because RMI timescales were very short, most of the required nursing information systems were not homegrown. Instead, systems designed for the U.S. private sector were transferred to the U.K. public sector with some limited adaptation.

> "The US systems were designed on the basis of assigning costs to individual patients based on the care given and the interventions undertaken and, as a consequence, this model was already encoded in the potential British systems" (Westrup, 1998:82).

As a result, "the nurses using (being used by) the system would have to follow the patterns of nursing care embodied in the system and based on the rather different U.S. health environment."

Because of their U.S. private sector origins, the transferred systems incorporated conceptions of nursing information needs, of links to other IT systems, of nursing processes, of nursing objectives and values, of nurse and health managers skills and knowledge, of nursing management approaches that were very different to the U.K. public sector reality.

For example, although the system incorporated rostering, "after nursing systems were implemented it was still common for nursing sisters to do the nursing roster at home as the computer system was found not to cater for the complexity of rostering in practice." As noted above, the system also fell down in the gap between the US-based conception of care planning as integral to nursing care and the UK reality that care planning was not generally done. The result was widespread total or partial failure of these systems:

"Hundreds of millions of pounds (and countless hours of people's time) were spent on information technology and systems introduced in virtually every hospital in Britain but it appears that few of them were successful by any criteria: complete implementation; actual use; or cost effectiveness" (Westrup, 1998:85).

Less than 30% of hospitals ever got their nursing information systems fully operational, and many of these were never fully used (HSMU, 1996).

CONCLUSIONS

A health care information system succeeds or fails – it is argued here – dependent on the degree of mismatch between the conceptions in that system's design and the realities into which it is introduced. We can assess that mismatch along seven main dimensions, described above in the ITPOSMO model. Given that failure is naturally more of a concern than success, and given that HCIS will fail more often than they succeed, three archetypal conception-reality gaps were presented which make failure more likely to occur:

- when healthcare information systems derived from hard rational models of organization meet a different behavioral reality;
- when HCIS derived from the private sector are transferred to public sector healthcare organizations;
- when HCIS derived from one country are transferred to another country, especially from an industrialized to a developing country.

Having provided an explanation for failure, the obvious question is: 'OK, so what do we do about it?'

Our starting point for any process of HCIS implementation must be analysis of the conception-reality gap. There is no straightforward method for analyzing the gap between current reality and the conceptions assumed within a proposed new healthcare information system. One approach – arising from Checkland's Soft Systems Methodology (Checkland and Scholes 1990) – is to undertake: a) analysis of current reality, and b) design of the new HCIS. In the case of both analysis and design, the seven ITPOSMO dimensions of change can be incorporated. Design can be used to expose inherent conceptions, so comparing reality and the design proposal along these dimensions will give an idea of the extent of change gaps (see Figure 1).

Soft systems methods often advocate recognition of gaps as potential changes, which can then be discussed in participative fora to identify those which are desirable and feasible. Where gaps are identified by participating stakeholder groups as both desirable and feasible changes to current reality, it may well be that they will be successfully implemented.

Gap Closure Techniques for Greater HCIS Success

In tandem, though, it will be valuable to make use of techniques which either a) prevent large gaps arising in the first place, or b) reduce those gaps once they have been identified. There are many ways in which gap prevention or gap reduction can be achieved. We present here just a sample of techniques that may help improve the success rate of HCIS initiatives.

Legitimizing and mapping organizational reality. An integral part of successful HCIS must be a proper understanding of current realities. This may often be difficult; for example, where rational paradigms dominate. In such situations, HCIS project leaders can help by "legitimizing reality" by encouraging participants to articulate the difference between rational, prescriptive models of what they should be doing and real depictions of what they are actually doing. Techniques for exposing and mapping organizational realities play a role here. Self- and third-party observation helps expose realities. Use of soft systems tools such as '"rich pictures" help map realities. Prototyping of HCIS helps both, particularly helping users to under-

Figure 1. The ITPOSMO Dimensions of Change for Health Care Information System Proposals

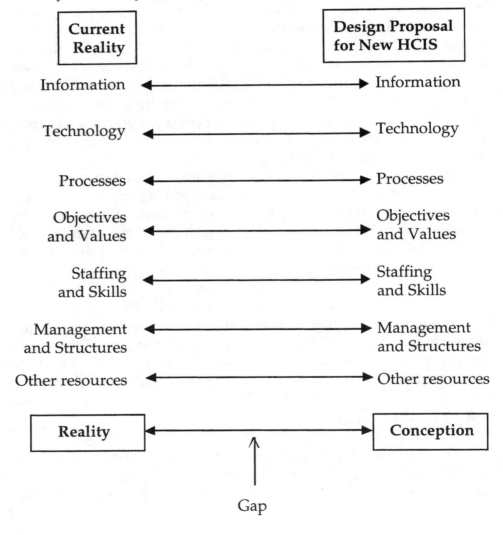

stand their real information needs. All of these techniques have been successfully applied to HCIS (Gillis, et al., 1994; Checkland and Holwell, 1998; Paré and Elam, 1998; Ballantine and Cunningham, 1999).

Reality-supporting not rationality-imposing applications. We can distinguish a continuum of healthcare applications, as illustrated in Figure 2. At one extreme, there are rationality-imposing applications such as decision support systems. These incorporate a whole series of assumptions about the presence of rational information, processes, objectives and values, management structures, etc. These rationalities must either be present in the organization as a precondition for successful implementation of this application, or they must be imposed. In many organizations, the introduction of such applications will not succeed because of the large gap between the application's required rationalities and current organizational realities. Hence, the problems found in introducing applications like DSS into many healthcare organizations (Vian, et al., 1993; Blake, et al., 1995; Edwards and Bushko, 1995; Ennals, et al., 1996).

At the other extreme, there are reality-supporting applications such as word processing. By comparison with rationality-imposing applications, reality-supporting applications require fewer conceptions to be met as preconditions or to be imposed. They can therefore work successfully in a wider variety of organizational environments. Hence, far from the gaze of those besotted by the "leading edge," the domination of word processing and e-mail as applications in health care settings (Young and Beswick, 1995; Smith and Harding, 1998).

Because they involve small conception-reality gaps, reality-supporting applications seem more likely to be successful and are therefore to be encouraged. Indeed, the importance of making healthcare applications as reality-supporting as possible explains the interest in HCIS features that more closely imitate reality, such as free text-based recording and search systems, pen and audio input, mobile computing, and integration of images into computerized medical records (Dayhoff, 1995; Laukkanen and Maier, 1995; Lincoln and Essin, 1995; Verhoosel, et al., 1998). Many HCIS may therefore have to become more technically sophisticated in order to become more reality-supporting and, hence, to integrate more easily into healthcare practice.

Customization to match realities. One general message is that whole health care sectors, organizations, and even individuals must continue to recognize, express and have satisfied their unique requirements. 'Customized' must therefore take precedence over "ready made," as has been found for a number of successful HCIS (Keijzer and Rodrigo, 1995; Miller, et al., 1995; Paré and Elam, 1998). In many cases, this will require national and/or sectoral and/or in-house HCIS capacities to be strengthened.

This will also affect selection of software vendors and developers. One key criterion will be their demonstrable willingness and ability to understand client contextual realities and to customize information systems accordingly. This finally has implications for the viability of healthcare organization client consortia, suggesting they will be relatively difficult to sustain (Gowing, 1994).

Change agents. The ITPOSMO model is a reminder that a focus on technology is too narrow and that HCIS must be seen as part of a multi-dimensional process of change. Healthcare IT professionals must therefore see themselves more as change agents (Markus and Benjamin, 1996). They may become facilitators by increasing the capacity of others to change, or they may become advocates who take responsibility for implementing change along the identified dimensions. In either case, their technology skills will be complemented by those of change management and of communication, negotiation and advocacy. To support this, there must be a change in the healthcare organization structures and management processes that deal with information systems, away from the old central IT unit model.

End-user development. Many of the gaps described in this chap-

Figure 2. Continuum of Health Care Applications

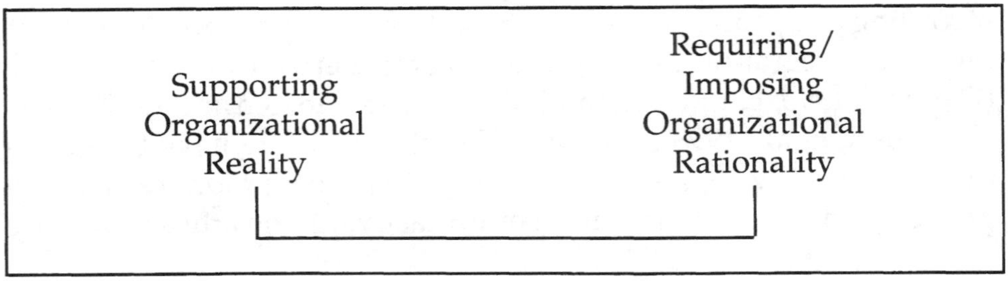

| Supporting Organizational Reality | Requiring/ Imposing Organizational Rationality |

ter are gaps between the context and assumptions of HCIS design and the context and assumptions of HCIS operation; that is, they are gaps between developers and users. One way to close these gaps almost entirely is through end-user development which vests all, or almost all, systems development roles in a single person. This will close the design—reality gaps of information needs, and of objectives and values. It can significantly reduce the money and time resource requirement, and end users are most unlikely to create unmanageable levels of change for themselves on the other ITPOSMO dimensions. As such, end-user development should greatly increase the chance of producing a successful health care information system, as has been found in practice (Edwards and Bushko, 1995).

Participation. Where end-user development is not feasible, conception-reality gaps can be reduced through participatory approaches that allow the world views of a range of stakeholders to be incorporated into HCIS design. This can particularly be used to close gaps along the objectives and values dimension. It can be difficult to combine or compromise between different hard, rational world views because such world views tend to be resistant to change. Nevertheless, participative approaches have proven to be the bedrock of successful HCIS projects in a wide variety of settings (Foltz, 1993; Rosenal, et al., 1995; Curry, 1998).

Hybridization. The previous three techniques all require some form of hybridization. Current IT professionals need to be hybridized into broader change agents who combine IS and IT skills with an understanding of the healthcare context and of change management. Current healthcare professionals need to be hybridized towards a broader skill set that includes an understanding of information systems and information technology (especially the latter for end-user developers). For example, training must aim to create "the informatics nurse" who can fully participate in HCIS initiatives (van Aulst and Springer, 1995).

Incrementalism. Where a major set of changes is planned as part of a new HCIS, breaking these down and introducing them only slowly and in an incremental manner will help to reduce the extent of any given change. This, in turn, will increase the likelihood of successful system introduction, as found in practice (Slater, 1996; Hoogewerf and Lowe, 1998).

Closing specific conception-reality gaps. The techniques already described are relatively generic to all ITPOSMO dimensions. However, techniques can also be employed to help close specific dimensional gaps. There are two main ways in which a gap between reality and proposal can be reduced: a) change current reality to make it closer to the HCIS design proposal, or b) change the HCIS design proposal to make it closer to reality. As an example of the former, staffing and skill realities can be brought closer to HCIS conceptions by hiring new temporary or permanent staff or through training schemes. Likewise, financial realities can be brought closer to HCIS conceptions by seeking new funding sources. Many public sector organizations are doing this through private finance initiatives under which private firms develop, own and operate the HCIS and are paid an annual fee over an agreed period for this service only if the service meets agreed criteria. Alternatively, HCIS conceptions can be brought closer to reality in both cases by reducing either the scale or scope of the HCIS design so that it requires fewer skilled staff or costs less to operate.

Freezing dimensions of change. Any dimension of the HCIS design proposal can be altered to make it smaller or simpler and thus closer to reality. This design alteration could go as far as making the new proposed design conceptions exactly match current reality along one particular dimension, by freezing that dimension. Going further, the proposal could match reality along several of the ITPOSMO dimensions. An example of the first would be freezing the technology dimension of change by not altering the IT but, instead, focusing change on the redesign of healthcare processes.

A Caveat on Techniques

Finally, though, we must issue a caveat about the techniques described above. We began by saying that a contingent approach to HCIS is required, but our focus in this chapter has been about contingency of information system *content* (the what) rather than information system *process* (the how). In other words, we have focused on matching the final information system to its context, but have not thought about matching IS implementation techniques to their contexts.

We must now do the latter in order to avoid presenting the listed techniques in a prescriptive, "cookbook" manner. We must therefore not say "participative approaches will always be part of successful HCIS implementation." Instead, we must say "first analyze the situation to see if these particular conditions hold; if they do, then participation is more likely to be of value; if they do not, then participation is less likely to be of value."

For example, user-participation techniques are unlikely to work well where:

- users lack information about participative techniques and about the new information system (information dimension);
- the objectives of senior staff are not to share power and the values of the organization are authoritarian and hierarchical (objectives and values dimension);
- users lack the skills and confidence necessary to engage in participative processes (staffing and skills dimension);
- the management style and organizational structures of the organization are highly centralized (management and structures dimension);
- the organization lacks the time and money to invest in participative approaches (other resources dimension).

From this example, it can be seen that we can apply the ITPOSMO model to the process of HCIS implementation. We can say that implementation techniques are less likely to work where there is a large gap between the conceptions inherent within those techniques and the realities of the organization in which you try to apply them. We can therefore use the conception-reality gap model to assess not just the feasibility of a particular HCIS design, but also the feasibility of particular HCIS implementation techniques.

Questions for Future Research

From the analysis above, three key questions arise for future research.

- *How and Why are Healthcare Managers Pressurized into High-Gain, High-Risk HCIS Initiatives?* Healthcare information systems with a larger conception-reality gap bring greater risks of failure, but they also typically promise greater organizational benefits from greater organizational change. Healthcare managers often find themselves in a dilemma, torn between one HCIS proposal that is revolutionary, high benefit and high risk, and another that is incremental, limited benefit and low risk. Future research can help understand the contextual – typically political – pressures that so often push managers to choose the former, leading to large, spectacular and very costly HCIS failures. Research is also needed to help managers identify options for modifying the political context, or, where modification is not possible, for reacting to that context in a lower-risk manner.

- *What Barriers Exist to Adoption of Common Best Practice Techniques?* The common "gap-closing" techniques described above, and their positive impact, are no secret. Future research should therefore focus not so much on describing common best practice techniques, but on analyzing the barriers to their adoption in healthcare organizations and on helping healthcare managers overcome those barriers. The question about hybridization, for example, is not "Does it deliver as a technique?" but "Why can't or don't HCIS projects use it more often?".

- *What Innovative Techniques Can be Adopted to Support HCIS Initiatives?* Common best practice techniques have been described, but a host of less well-known or less well-tried techniques exist that can close conception-reality gaps and can improve the success rate of healthcare information systems. Further research is required to identify, assess and disseminate such techniques. One example might be a tacit knowledge/informal information systems approach that seeks to expose and support the tacit knowledge that is key to many healthcare organization functions, as used in the "soft network" approach of Yorkshire Health Associates in the UK (Hastings, 1996).

REFERENCES

Alendahl, K., Timpka, T. and Sjöberg, C. (1995). Computerized knowledge bases in primary health care, in: *Medinfo '95*, R.A. Greenes, H.E. Peterson and D.J. Protti (eds), Healthcare Computing and Communications Canada, Edmonton, 917-921.

Anderson, J.G. (1997). Clearing the way for physicians' use of clinical information systems, *Communications of the ACM*, 40(8), 83-90.

Ballantine, J. and Cunningham, N. (1999). Strategic information systems planning: Applying private sector frameworks in UK public healthcare, in: *Reinventing Government in the Information Age*, R.B. Heeks (ed.), Routledge, London, 293-311.

Beynon-Davies, P. (1995). Information systems 'failure': The case of the London Ambulance Service's Computer Aided Despatch project, *European Journal of Information Systems*, 4, 171-184.

Blake, J., Carter, M., O'Brien-Pallas, L. and McGillis-Hill, L. (1995). A surgical process management tool, in: *Medinfo '95*, R.A. Greenes, H.E. Peterson and D.J. Protti (eds.), Healthcare Computing and Communications Canada, Edmonton, 527-531.

Brennan, P.F. and Ripich, S. (1994). Use of a home-care computer network by persons with AIDS, *International Journal of Technology Assessment in Health Care*, 10(2), 258-272.

Butler, R. (1991). *Designing Organizations*, Routledge, New York.

Checkland, P.B. and Holwell, S. (1998). *Information, Systems and Information Systems*, Wiley, Chichester, UK.

Checkland, P.B. and Scholes, J. (1990). *Soft Systems Methodology in Action*, Wiley, Chichester, UK.

Coiera, E. (1997). *Guide to Medical Informatics, the Internet and Telemedicine*, Chapman and Hall, London.

Curry, P. (1998). Big hospital systems: Problems in implementation, in: *Current Perspectives in Healthcare Computing 1998*, B. Richards (ed.), BJHC, Weybridge, UK, 3-7.

Davies, C.A. (1997). The information infrastructure approach, paper presented at conference on '*Public Sector Management in the Next Century*', 29 June-2 July, University of Manchester, Manchester, UK.

Davies, H.T.O. and Nutley, S.M. (1999). The rise and rise of evidence in health care, *Public Money and Management*, 19(1), 9-16.

Dayhoff, R.E., Kirin, G., Pollock, S. and Todd, S. (1995). Data capture workstations, scanned forms, and pen-based systems for clinician use, in: *Medinfo '95*, R.A. Greenes, H.E. Peterson and D.J. Protti (eds.), Healthcare Computing and Communications Canada, Edmonton, p1679.

Dhillon, G. (1998). *The Clinical Information System: A Case of Misleading Design Decisions*, Case 1-98-IT06, Idea Group Publishing, Hershey, PA.

Dodd, W. and Fortune, J. (1995). An electronic patient record project in the United Kingdom: Can it succeed?, in: *Medinfo '95*, R.A. Greenes, H.E. Peterson and D.J. Protti (eds), Healthcare Computing and Communications Canada, Edmonton, 301-304.

Dusserre, P., Allaert, F.A. and Dusserre, L. (1995). The emergence of international telemedicine: No ready-made solutions exist, in: *Medinfo '95*, R.A. Greenes, H.E. Peterson and D.J. Protti (eds.), Healthcare Computing and Communications Canada, Edmonton, 1475-1478.

Edwards, G.A. and Bushko, R.G. (1995). Business modeling tools for managing decision support systems, in: *Medinfo '95*, R.A. Greenes, H.E. Peterson and D.J. Protti (eds), Healthcare Computing and Communications Canada, Edmonton, 1005-1008.

Ennals, R., Pound, H., Graydon, P. and Sercombe, J. (1996). An assessment of information technology in three health service settings, in: *Creative Computing in Health and Social Care*, F. Yates (ed.), John Wiley, Chichester, UK, 39-54.

Foltz, A.M. (1993). Modeling technology transfer in health information systems, *International Journal of Technology Assessment in Health Care*, 9(3), 346-359.

Gillis, P.A., Booth, H., Graves, J.R., Fehlauer, C.S. and Soller, J. (1994). Translating traditional principles of system development into a process for designing clinical information systems, *International Journal of Technology Assessment in Health Care*, 10(2), 235-248.

Gowing, W. (1994). Operational systems, in: *Information Management in Health Services*, J. Keen (ed.), Open University Press, Buckingham, UK, 31-49.

Greaves, P.J. (1998). Nurses' knowledge of patient information security in healthcare information systems — a cause for concern, in: *Current Perspectives in Healthcare Computing 1998*, B. Richards (ed.), BJHC, Weybridge, UK, 77-84.

Guah, M.W. (1998). *Evaluation and Analysis of Multimedia Information System Design and Implementation at the Coloscopy Unit of St. James University Hospital, Leeds, UK*, M.Sc. dissertation, School of Management, UMIST, Manchester.

Hastings, C. (1996). *The New Organization*, McGraw-Hill, London.

Health Committee (1995). *London's Ambulance Service*, Report HC20,

Her Majesty's Stationery Office, London.

Heeks, R.B. and Bhatnagar, S.C. (1999). Understanding success and failure in information age reform, in: *Reinventing Government in the Information Age*, R.B. Heeks (ed.), Routledge, London, 49-74.

Heeks, R.B. and Davies, A. (1999). Different approaches to information age reform, in: *Reinventing Government in the Information Age*, R.B. Heeks (ed.), Routledge, London, 22-48.

Hoogewerf, J. and Lowe, S. (1998). Partnership in practice: A collaborative approach to progressing primary healthcare team systems, in: *Current Perspectives in Healthcare Computing 1998*, B. Richards (ed.), BJHC, Weybridge, UK, 51-58.

HSMU (1996). *The Evaluation of the NHS Resource Management Programme in England*, Health Services Management Unit, University of Manchester, Manchester.

IMG (1996). *HISS Project Probe Reviews of Addenbrooke's Trust, James Paget Hospital Trust, Norfolk and Norwich Healthcare Trust and West Suffolk Hospitals Trust*, Information Management Group, NHS Executive, Winchester.

Ireland, M.C. and Regan, B.G. (1995). General practice medical records: Is coding appropriate?, in: *Medinfo '95*, R.A. Greenes, H.E. Peterson and D.J. Protti (eds.), Healthcare Computing and Communications Canada, Edmonton, 47-50.

Isaacs, S. (1995). The human-data interface: A comparison of the cognitive style of the IT department with that of the management, in: *Medinfo '95*, R.A. Greenes, H.E. Peterson and D.J. Protti (eds.), Healthcare Computing and Communications Canada, Edmonton, 789-791.

James, G. (1997). IT fiascoes...and how to avoid them, *Datamation* November. http://www.datamation.com/PlugIn/issues/1997/november/11disas.html.

Jayasuriya, R. (1995). Health care informatics from theory to practice: lessons from a case study in a developing country, in: *Medinfo '95*, R.A. Greenes, H.E. Peterson and D.J. Protti (eds), Healthcare Computing and Communications Canada, Edmonton, 1603-1607.

Keen, J. (ed.) (1994a). *Information Management in Health Services*, Open University Press, Buckingham, UK.

Keen, J. (1994b). Should the National Health Service have an information strategy?, *Public Administration*, 72, 33-53.

Keijzer, J.C. and Rodrigo, S.G. (1995). Three Dutch hospitals, in: *Transforming Health Care Through Information*, N.M. Lorenzi, R.T. Riley, M.J. Ball and J.V. Douglas (eds.), Springer-Verlag, New York, 391-399.

Korac-Boisvert, N. and Kouzmin, A. (1995). Transcending soft-core IT disasters in public sector organizations, *Information Infrastructure and Policy*, 4(2), 131-161.

Laukkanen, E. and Maier, M. (1995). Design and implementation of an electronic point-of-contact oncology clinical record, in: *Medinfo '95*, R.A. Greenes, H.E. Peterson and D.J. Protti (eds.), Healthcare Computing and Communications Canada, Edmonton, 317-318.

Lincoln, T.L. and Essin, D.J. (1995). A document processing architecture for electronic medical records, in: *Medinfo '95*, R.A. Greenes, H.E. Peterson and D.J. Protti (eds.), Healthcare Computing and Communications Canada, Edmonton, 227-230.

Markus, M.L. and Benjamin, R.I. (1996). Change agentry – the next frontier, *MIS Quarterly*, 20(4), 385-407.

McDaniel, J.G., Moehr, J.R. and Müller, H.A. (1995). Impediments to developing wide area networks in health care, in: *Medinfo '95*, R.A. Greenes, H.E. Peterson and D.J. Protti (eds), Healthcare Computing and Communications Canada, Edmonton, 1491-1495.

Miller, E.T., Wieckert, K.E., Fagan, L.M. and Musen, M.A. (1995). The development of a controlled medical terminology: identification, collaboration, and customization, in: *Medinfo '95*, R.A. Greenes, H.E. Peterson and D.J. Protti (eds), Healthcare Computing and Communications Canada, Edmonton, 148-152.

Neumann, P.J., Parente, S.T. and Paramore, L.C. (1996). Potential savings from using information technology applications in health care in the United States, *International Journal of Technology Assessment in Health Care*, 12(3), 425-435.

Page, D., Williams, P. and Boyd, D. (1993). *Report of the Public Inquiry into the London Ambulance Service*, South West Thames Regional Health Authority, London.

Paré, G. and Elam, J.J. (1998). Introducing information technology in the clinical setting, *International Journal of Technology Assessment in Health Care*, 14(2), 331-343.

Poulymenakou, A. and Holmes, A. (1996). A contingency framework for the investigation of information systems failure, *European Journal of Information Systems*, 5, 34-46.

Raghupathi, W. (1997). Health care information systems, *Communications of the ACM*, 40(8), 81-82.

Roberts, A. and Garnett, D. (1998). Standard generalised mark-up language for electronic patient records, in: *Current Perspectives in Healthcare Computing 1998*, B. Richards (ed.), BJHC, Weybridge, UK, 249-255.

Rosenal, T., Patterson, R., Wakefield, S., Zuege, D. and Lloyd-Smith, G. (1995). Physician involvement in hospital information system selection: A success story, in: *Medinfo '95*, R.A. Greenes, H.E. Peterson and D.J. Protti (eds), Healthcare Computing and Communications Canada, Edmonton, 554-558.

Slater, E. (1996). Slowly but surely, *Health Service Journal*, 17 October, 8-9.

Smith, M.F. and Harding, G. (1998). Computer user attitudes and fluency, in: *Current Perspectives in Healthcare Computing 1998*, B. Richards (ed.), BJHC, Weybridge, UK, 310-316.

Steimann, F. (1995). A case against logic, in: *Medinfo '95*, R.A. Greenes, H.E. Peterson and D.J. Protti (eds), Healthcare Computing and Communications Canada, Edmonton, 989-993.

van Aulst, E.H. and Springer, H. (1995). The training of the informatics nurse: An intermediary between the discipline of nursing and the developers of information systems, in: *Medinfo '95*, R.A. Greenes, H.E. Peterson and D.J. Protti (eds.), Healthcare Computing and Communications Canada, Edmonton, 1344-1348.

Verhoosel, J.P.C., de Bruin, B. and Oldenkamp, J.H. (1998). Mobile data applications in hospitals, in: *Current Perspectives in Healthcare Computing 1998*, B. Richards (ed.), BJHC, Weybridge, UK, 397-403.

Vian, T., Verjee, S., and Siegrist, R.B. (1993). Decision support systems in health care, *International Journal of Technology Assessment in Health Care*, 9(3), 369-379.

Vogt, W.B., Bhattacharya, I., Kupor, S., Yoshikawa, A. and Nakahara, T. (1996). Technology and staffing in Japanese university hospitals: Government versus private, *International Journal of Technol-*

ogy Assessment in Health Care, 12(1), 93-103.

Westrup, C. (1998). What's in information technology?, in: *Implementation and Evaluation of Information Systems in Developing Countries*, C. Avgerou (ed.), Asian Institute of Technology, Bangkok, 77-91.

Young, A.J. and Beswick, K.B.J. (1995). Decision support in the United Kingdom for general practice, in: *Medinfo '95*, R.A. Greenes, H.E. Peterson and D.J. Protti (eds.), Healthcare Computing and Communications Canada, Edmonton, 1025-1029.

Chapter VI

The Use of Artificial Intelligence Techniques and Applications in the Medical Domain

Adi Armoni
Tel-Aviv College of Management, Israel

In recent years we have witnessed sweeping developments in information technology. Currently, the most promising and interesting domain seemed to be the artificial intelligence. Within this field we see now a growing interest in the medical applications. The purpose of this article is to present a general review of the main areas of artificial intelligence and its applications to the medical domain. The review will focus on artificial intelligence applications to radiology, robotically-operated surgical procedures and different kinds of expert systems.

INTRODUCTION

The true challenge of artificial intelligence lies in the duplication of the mental capacities of ordinary people, such as vision and natural language (the language of speech as opposed to computer language). These actions may seem simple and natural to most of us, but in order to express them on the computer we will require the most complicated algorithms. "The fact that we are able to carry out the complicated act of vision at minimal effort, compared to complicated acts of multiplication, is almost an error of evolution ...." (Nilsen, 1990).

Indeed, research and development in the field of artificial intelligence mainly focus on the attempt to imitate "basic" human actions such as: speech recognition, vision, and various mechanical actions (assembly, analysis, dividing samples into petri dishes, storing professional knowledge and producing it when required expertise).

There are different definitions of artificial intelligence, Charniak's definition (Charniak, McDermott, 1989) : "Artificial intelligence is studying mental capacities through the use of computerized models." It is easier to understand the potential value of artificial intelligence when we confront it with human intelligence. According to Kaplan (1994), artificial intelligence has a number of clear commercial advantages over natural intelligence:

- Artificial intelligence is more "steady," as it does not depend on workers' rotation, nor is it based on their memory. It ensures that as long as the software and hardware are in good shape the use we create will not change.
- Artificial intelligence ensures easy distribution and duplication. The process of transferring knowledge from one person to another is long and complicated, and it is almost impossible to duplicate human experts, unlike the duplication of computerized systems.
- As artificial intelligence is computerized technology, it is consequential and accurate (of course to the extent that the information fed into the database is consequential and accurate), compared to natural intelligence which is founded on the lack of stability of the human expert.
- The actions and decisions received from computerized systems are easy to document by following the stages of their receipt and therefore it is possible to study and examine them. On the other hand, the human expert is capable of drawing a conclusion, while at a later stage he will be unable to explain the sequence of deductions leading to this conclusion.

Compared to the advantages of artificial intelligence mentioned above, natural intelligence also has a few striking advantages:

- Natural intelligence is creative, compared to the rigidity characterizing artificial intelligence. Human beings possess the ability to acquire knowledge and draw conclusions, whereas artificial intelligence adapted to the requirements of the system, is generally fixed and well planned.

- Human beings are able to make immediate use of information received through the senses, whereas the computerized system requires symbolic signal processing.
- The most important advantage is the ability of human beings to integrate relevant knowledge from a number of fields and expertise and coordinate this in order to find the solution to a certain problem. Compared to this ability, the computerized systems are merely based on narrow, centralized information.

THE CONCEPT OF KNOWLEDGE IN ARTIFICIAL INTELLIGENCE

In the field of information systems, a distinction is usually made between data, information and knowledge. In data terms it is common to refer to strings of numeric or alpha-numeric values which in themselves are of no importance.

These strings may include numeric values or facts that must be processed.

On the other hand, information is a group of facts which is organized and processed in a manner that is significant to the person who receives it.

Information has many definitions, one of the best is by Turban (1995) "information includes all the clear and the concealed limits connected with a certain object, for the activities and the interactions of this object. The information also includes specific heuristic rules and procedures of drawing conclusions, all of them connected with the situation one wishes to model and which pertain to the object in question.

The facts, information and knowledge may be classified in accordance with the extent to which they are abstract and according to their quantity (Figure 1) when the information is abstract to the highest degree and exists in the smallest quantity.

MAIN FIELDS OF RESEARCH AND APPLICATION

During recent years we witness a great interest and progress in implementing artificial intelligence techniques dealing with processing and retrieving medical knowledge, diagnostic tolls, decision support and expert systems, and computerized supplies to perform

Figure 1: Mesuring the Quantity and Abstraction of Knowledge, Information and Facts

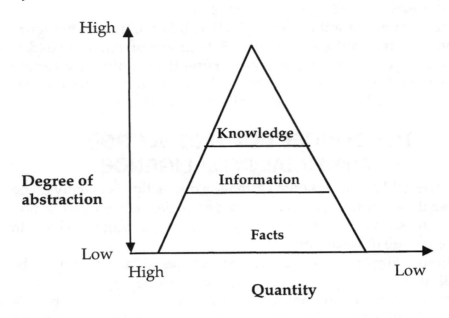

an invasive procedures.

We will discuss and demonstrate the up-to-date research topics and application of artificial intelligence. Among those topics we can find techniques of robotics, computerized vision, expert systems, speech recognition, neural networks, etc.

ROBOTICS

We must remember that it is very difficult to define and execute actions that are not founded on explicit algorithm. For example, although it seems as if housework is a simple act, and not as complicated as powerful precision welding, from the robot's point of view, the latter is much easier, for the part arrives exactly at the right time at the right place, and all that remains is to carry out the welding.

On the other hand, housework requires the robot to see and understand everything around him. He must distinguish between the piano and the bed, know where the sheets are (they are placed differently each time), etc.

The main problem still remains the ability to transfer the "human feeling and perception" to the robot. If we recall that the human hand is capable of holding a piece of paper in various ways without creasing it, a wet glass without letting it slide, or crack a hard nut, we will understand how hard it is to impart these natural talents to an artificial limb which has no feeling and understanding of the meaning of the action (Amato, 1992). The main medical applications of robotics focus on three fields:

Surgery -including laparoscopic cholecystectomy (Ganger, 1996). Introducing miniature robots via the blood vessels in microsurgery (Wickham, 1994) accurate and swift prostatectomy, whereby the robot carrying out the section is placed via an image obtained from the ultrasound device (Ng et al, 1993).

Surgery to replace the hip bone, when the robot assists in the entire process of planning, locating, directing and carrying out the surgery. A three-dimensional form of the area of the operation, together with the geometric basis of knowledge, allow the robot to direct the surgeon and automatically carry out the required drilling and cutting at the optimal location (Matesen, 1993).

Laboratories — Analysis of genetic sequences and dividing blood samples into serological tests, when the robot uses the division of the material into samples in a systematically, accurate and efficient manner, prevents human errors and drastically (up to 50%) reduces the time of work (Caillat, et al., 1995; Wilson, 1995).

Locating and conveying of medical equipment —After a number of years in which the artificial intelligence technology has been implemented at various levels of sophistication at industrial warehouses, these applications have also arrived at medical locations. The system that was developed enables the computerized locating of drugs at pharmacies and conveying them to the party ordering them (Landis, 1993). Automatic conveying of medical equipment from warehouses to hospital wards and departments (Tadano, 1995).

COMPUTERIZED VISION

This is defined as an addition to artificial intelligence, capable of monitoring and analyzing visual information received from various sensors (video cameras, electronic scanners, etc.) and adding it to the information existing in the system. The recognition technique is based on the analysis of the received input and verifying it against the data stored in the computer's database. Computerized vision uses complicated techniques and mathematical algorithms, most of which are based on the techniques of pattern recognition (Turban, 1995). The information analyzed by the system may, for example, be used for controlling a robot's movement, monitoring the speed of a conveyor belt, and automatic quality control of items under production.

There is a wide range of applications of computerized vision in the medical field. We will divide these applications into three main groups:

Pathological diagnosis — Through automatic input of data from the mammography machine (Vyborny and Giger, 1996) or oral lesions according to direct input from the computerized tomography instrument (Brooks, 1995). The application of computerized vision is also presented for automatic follow-up and classification of the size of the pituitary microadenoma (Cannavo, et al., 1992), and on-line cytological diagnosis according to the data supplied by a needle introduced into the suspected tumor (Wolberg, et. al., 1995).

Recognition of the structure of materials —Comparing the molecular structure with the computerized database to the molecular structure seen by the computerized system makes it possible to recognize the chemical and physical structure of the material (Heiden, et. al., 1995), or changes in the mineral bone composition (Robertson, 1996), or automatic location of materials through the identification of the amino-acid structure (Ficher, et al., 1995).

Graph analysis—Mostly through techniques of pattern recognition for the purpose of comparing graphs from the computerized data base with the input values received from the system/the medical instrument. There are leading applications in the field of retina lesions through the analysis of the results of fields of vision tests (Martin, 1995), diagnosis and recognition of phases in the course of sleep through the analysis of output received from the EEG instrument (Hasan et. al., 1995), or studying the cortical vision mechanisms (Miyashita et. al., 1995).

EXPERT SYSTEMS

General

This is the artificial intelligence field with the largest number of applications. The expert systems are very important because of their inherent potential to replace experts in fields in which it is expensive to find people who possess the knowledge.

In these systems we endeavor to learn the expertise of the person (or in professional language: to extract the expert's knowledge) and integrate this knowledge in the computerized system's database. Unlike the computerized systems familiar to all of us, which include a database and a models base, in the expert systems we find an additional module called "knowledge base." In this module the information extracted from the human expert will be stored.

Striking expert systems are to be found in the medical diagnostic field, electronics and computers (for example: for examination and automatic location of failures in electronic components).

The most frequently mentioned and described system is no doubt the **Mycin** (Buchanan and Shortliffe, 1984) system, developed at Stanford University in the early seventies.

The purpose of the project was described as the development and application of a system that would point out the best way of treating a patient suspected of suffering from an infectious disease. This system identifies the virus (the most likely one) causing the infection, and in accordance with what is found, as mentioned above, it recommends the best method of treatment.

In the early eighties an expert system was developed at Pittsburgh University in the field of internal medicine. This system, called **Internist -1** enables the physician to carry out an accurate differentiated diagnostic process (Miller, et. al., 1992).

For the diagnosis and treatment of the group of glaucoma diseases, an expert system was developed in the early eighties at Rutgers University, called **Casnet** (Kulikowski and Weiss, 1992).

This expert system, like the Mycin system, contributed significantly to the development of expert systems, basing themselves on the expert systems generator called **Expert** (Weiss et. al. 1992).

With the use and the contribution to the development of this generator which is independent in the field of application, the systems created a very powerful tool for the definition of additional medical expert systems.

Neomycin (Clancey and Letsinger, 1991) and **Caduceus** (Pople, 1985) belong to the second generation of expert systems. In this generation of expert systems, stronger emphasis is placed on the presentation of the cause and effects of the disease, the control procedures have become more complicated, and much work was invested in the addition of information and its reorganization in the data base of the systems. Indeed, the **Neomycin** system is an improved version of the **Mycin** system and the **Caduceus** system is an improved version of the **Internist -1** system.

There are still reasons, some of them objective (such as the problem to include huge quantities of information, accurate and consistent extraction of the expert's knowledge), and others subjective (the physician's fear of basing himself on computerized systems), which prevent the large-scale use of these systems.

However, we are quite certain that the progress of medical science and the huge quantities of information to which the physician is exposed will oblige those occupied in medicine to use the computerized systems in the diagnostic process. It is quite clear that a physician who uses an expert system in his field will be more consistent and methodical in the process of diagnosis than a physician who operates without such a system.

Because the expert systems are so important in the application of artificial intelligence in medicine, I shall provide a more detailed description of four of the most famous systems surveyed above.

The MYCIN System for Diagnosis and Treatment of Infectious Diseases

This is the best known and most often described expert system among medical systems. This project was already started at Stanford University in 1972 and was based on the cooperation between a team composed of computer scientists and people treating infectious diseases at this university's school of medicine.

The target of the research was defined as the development and application of a system that would provide a guideline for the best way to treat a patient suspected of suffering from an infectious disease. The development of this project was considered very important, as the decisions regarding treatment must often be carried out under conditions of partial lack of certainty regarding the identification of the virus causing the infection. It is possible to make a perfect diagnosis of a large part of the infectious diseases, but only very rarely can the treating physician "allow himself" to wait a few days to receive the results of the lab tests (Buchanan BG & Shortliffe EH, 1997).

The information available to the physician at the stage in which the recommended treatment must be determined is mainly based on the patient's medical history, present symptoms and initial results of the lab tests. On the basis of these facts and the knowledge of experts of infectious diseases extracted from the experts which is presented in the database of the system, we expect MYCIN to carry out the following two stages:

- To identify the virus (the most likely one) causing the infection.
- To recommend, on the basis of the finding mentioned in section A above, the best manner of treatment.

As we mentioned above, one of the aims of the system is to discuss the subject of missing information and lack of certainty. In order to deal with the problem of lack of certainty, the term "certainty factor" was developed. At each and every stage of the process of diagnosis, we encounter a number of assumptions vying with each other as to the explanation of the phenomenon (attention: there is not only one single assumption, for in that case there is no lack of certainty at all).

The system attaches a numeric value to each of the assumptions describing the amount of certainty (strength) with which this assumption supports the explanation of the phenomenon.

This number value fluctuates between 1, i.e., absolute certainty regarding the quality of the assumption, through 0, indicating total lack of information or, alternatively, an identical amount of proof in favor of and against the assumption, and including 1, which indicates the assumption in no way supports the explanation of the phenomenon (absolute certainty that the assumption is not correct).

That is why this system is so important as a landmark in the development of expert systems in the medical field.

The INTERNIST 1 System for the Diagnosis
of Diseases in Internal Medicine

This system was developed at Pittsburgh University in the early eighties (Miller, et. al., 1992). From the beginning the emphasis in this system as placed on the correct application of the differentiated diagnostic process, based on a process of creating a set of diagnoses supporting at different levels of clarity findings that came to light in the clinical tests or the lab tests. At a later stage the tests whose clarity is at a lower level than the others will be eliminated from this set of tests.

We will distinguish between two kinds of entity in the database of the system: the diseases on the one hand, and the findings on the other hand. This database includes 500 diseases and about 3550 findings. For each disease a list of findings was defined that are known to be connected with this disease (this list was called "the profile of the disease" by the developers). The internist -1 system was developed in order to provide the physician with a tool to carry out an analysis in the field of internal medicine.

The diagnosis in this system is founded on two processes. One of them examines what findings are present or absent, and on the strength of these two facts creates a group of possible diseases. The other develops the heuristics that create the questions for the person using it for the purpose of obtaining additional information (clinical or lab tests) to enable support of the chosen diagnosis. At this stage a numeric value is attached to each diagnosis, stating the extent to which the findings support the diagnosis. In general, findings that are in the "profile of the disease" and were found with the patient add a positive value in support of the diagnosis; on the other hand, findings that are found in the "profile of the disease," but were not found with the patient, derogate from the credibility of the diagnosis.

Once the iterative process of the diagnosis is completed, the diagnosis which obtained the highest number of points from among the set of initial diagnoses is chosen.

CASNET System for the Diagnosis and Treatment of the Glaucoma Diseases Group

This system was developed in the early eighties at Rutgers University. It supplies methodology for expressing the interaction between the pathophysiological situations and the development of the disease.

The best known application of this methodology deals with the group of glaucoma diseases (Kulikowski and Weiss, 1992).

The system deals both with the process of diagnosis and the process of curing the diseases. Three kinds of objects are defined in Casnet findings (called observations), pathophysiological situations and categories of diseases. Each of these objects may be in one of the following situations: correct/confirmed, wrong/unconfirmed or unknown/undefined. It is possible to refer to the three kinds of objects as if they are on three separate levels, inter-linked and linked to the other levels through the situations described above.

The findings are the direct evidence pertaining to the patient (pain, lab test results). The pathophysiological situations are the summary of events that are different from ordinary behavior. These situations describe internal developments which may be presumed to take place in the patient's body, but cannot be observed externally. The pathophysiological situations are linked to each other through "response creating" relations. There may, of course, be more than one reason for a certain situation and this situation may create more than one response.

CASNET, like other expert systems in the medical field, fluctuates between examination of the patient's present problem on the strength of existing facts, and the need to ask additional clarifying questions (which are indeed asked in the course of the process).

The examination of the CASNET system's validity was carried out in various ways (Kulikowski and Weiss, 1992). However, the most comprehensive empirical test of the system's validity was carried out by linking the system to the Onet computer system used jointly by a number of eye clinics in the USA. In this test the system was examined on a large number of patients, and a 75% success rate was reported in the diagnosis of serious and complicated cases of glaucoma.

PIP System for the Diagnosis of Kidney Diseases

The PIP (Present Illness Program) system was developed by a group of scientists from MIT, together with colleagues from Tufts University's School of Medicine. The true purpose of the development of this system was the attempt to carry out a computerized simulation of the decision-making process in the medical field.

The researchers estimated on the strength of Elstein's work (Elstein, et. al., 1992) that human experts are very pressed in the process of creating hypotheses pertaining to the patient's situation, and do not have enough patience to examine a broad spectrum of facts, deduct the hypotheses with the highest probability and continue to raise additional questions on the strength of these hypotheses.

The medical field in which the PIP system was developed deals with the diagnosis of various kinds of kidney disease

The system includes sets of diseases and findings. There are characteristics for the various findings, and values were attached to these characteristics. For example, edema is a finding whose characteristics may be: presence (yes/no), location (legs, hands, etc.) rate of seriousness (accompanied by pain, not accompanied by pain), etc.

The information pertaining to each disease is organized in a frame which includes a number of cells. For each disease a status is defined that may be active, semi-active or not active. The group of diseases with the active status of course constitutes the group on which discussion must focus. Work in the system starts by feeding a group of general findings pertaining to the patient into the computer: age, sex, main symptoms. For each disease a group of "stimulant findings" is defined. In the event such a finding is received, the disease becomes active.

However, in addition to the list of "stimulant findings," there is an additional list of findings that may be related to the various diseases (not with absolute certainty and therefore they are not "stimulant findings"). Each time additional findings are received, a calculation is made of scores and rating of all the stimulant and semi-stimulant diseases. The score process is very complicated and actually consists of two parts :

- **Matching score**: assesses the extent to which the new findings match those that were anticipated, in accordance with the pattern characterizing the disease. This score actually assesses the extent to which our expectations from the new findings were realized.
- **The binding score**: assesses the extent to which the disease constitutes an accurate explanation of the findings received, i.e., what proportion of the findings received is explained by the disease. After evaluation of the active and semi-active hypotheses the discussion naturally focuses on hypotheses that have the highest score. At this stage the system (in accordance with the value of the score) decides whether to ask for additional evidence or point to the hypotheses that have the highest probability (Pauker, et al., 1996).

SPEECH RECOGNITION

This application includes the recognition of vocal input by the computer, i.e., the computer recognizes and decodes the vocal input and acts in accordance with what is said on it. The main applications that exist in medicine at present are in the field of assisting the disabled suffering from serious problems of movement (Taylor, et al., 1993), by issuing instructions to the robot with their voice; actions such as steering the wheelchair, operating electrical appliances and phone-dialing are carried out (Bach, 1995). There are also reports about experiments aimed at assisting and guiding reading for those suffering from serious eye problems. This guidance is carried out by comparing the written text with the text read by the patient and extending vocal feedback to the patient (Buning and Hanzlik, 1995). Medical applications are also found whose purpose it is to reduce the time of activity and the errors in printing diagnoses. For example, diagnosis of x-ray results by the physician and reading them out to the computer (La Fianza, et al., 1995; Mrosek, et al., 1995). This is based on a vocabulary of 20,000-30,000 words the physician will use. In a test (Buning and Hanzlik, 1995) carried out on the subject of the diagnosis of oral x-rays, it was reported that the time of treatment in the diagnosis according to voice recognition was 671 seconds, compared to merely 182 seconds in ordinary dictation to the typist.

This huge time gap is one of the reasons for the present failure of technology, which still requires adjusting the system to each user (through studying his voice) and is based on a closed vocabulary.

NEURAL NETWORKS

The name "neural networks" refers to two directions of research that are linked to each other: one deals with building models for components and functions of the nervous system in animals attempting to obtain maximum adjustment of anatomical and physiological facts. The other focuses on examining theoretical-mathematical computational systems with a structure that recalls a group of neurons.

The models in the first field refer to different levels in the nervous system:

- Single nerve cell—properties of the electric transmission in it, ionic ducts activity and the action organism of synopsis (Agmon and Segev, 1995, Powers, 1995).
- Group of nerve cells with emphasis on collective phenomena of their action (42, 43).
- Areas of the brain and mental functions such as memory (Zipser et al., 1993; Ruppin, et al., 1995).

There are also various functional emphases, for example in the ability of a model to show pathological situations or adaptation (Hinton, 1992). Moreover, in the past years an effort was made to develop and build network hardware, i.e., electronic chips whose activity is based on a large number of simple processing units, a kind of neuron, instead of a powerful and fast central processor, existing in the present computers. Together with the ripening of the neural networks theory, the applications increase (Armoni, 1998).

The potential for use is vast and includes almost any kind of information processing: statistical classification and regression, signal processing, image processing, etc. (Regia, 1993).

In this respect the computational nerve networks must be considered part of the entire range of statistical methods and modern information processing tools.

From the physician's point of view, neural networks may assist in day-to-day work and even in medical management at the department level.

Unlike expert systems based on rules drafted by professionals, neural networks can process unprocessed information: numeric results of tests, EEG, ECG (Edenbrandt et. al., 1995), imaging (Miller, et al., 1992; Cappini, et al., 1992). They are capable of finding complicated statistical correlation hidden even from the expert's eyes, and thus improve the standard of diagnosis (Boon and Kok, 1995; Cohen, et al., 1995).

Furthermore, the networks are capable of recognizing the relevant facts for diagnosis and prognosis from among tens and sometimes hundreds of possible variables (Baxt,1992). This makes it possible to shorten the diagnostic process, save on tests and efficiently manage the limited resources available to the medical field.

We would like to mention, as an example, improvement in the prediction of the natural history of disease and treatment of the mentally ill (Modai, 1993), cancer patients (Burke, 1996, Kappen and Neijt, 1995), and prediction of the period of time in which the patients will have to remain in intensive care (Tu and Guerriere, 1995).

Increasing attention is already being paid at present to computational neural networks, by intelligent use they will be able to improve activity in the field of medicine.

DISCUSSION

During the last years we witnessed a growing trend of utilizing a variety of artificial intelligence techniques in the medical domain. Those applications cover all branches of medicine, from diagnosis to the performance and interpretation of computerized tomography and end in numerous invasive procedures. The article supplies a comprehensive and up-to-date overview of artificial intelligence use in medicine, and points out the most promising trends and directions of evolution.

Since the greatest advance was in the field of retrieving, encoding, and using the expert's knowledge in knowledge-based systems, we found it proper to emphasize and examine more precisely part of our review on the expert systems domain.

It is clear to distinguish the two main advantages of the artificial intelligence over the human intelligence. The first is stemming from the consistent and accurate way of handling huge amount of data concerning symptoms, and disease and the continuous update, storage and accurate retrieve of this information (for example, expert systems, and all kinds of knowledge bases attached to diagnostic instruments).

The second advantage is related to the opportunity of focused and accurate performance of surgical and invasive procedures, while minimizing the dependence in the expert's skills.

The author has no doubt that in the next two to three years, the use of artificial intelligence will dramatically increase since the human brain and skills are not able to handle competitively the enormous quantity of data, information and knowledge, and to gain the full advantage of the high performance diagnostic appliances, but using the mentioned above artificial skills and techniques.

REFERENCES

Agmon-Shir H & Segev I. (1995). Signal delay and input synchronization in passive dendritic structures. *J Neurophysiol*, 70, 2066-2085.

Amato, I. (1992). In search of the human touch. *Science*, 258, 1436-1437.

Armoni, A.(1998). Utilization of Neural Networks in Medical Diagnosis, M.D. *Computing*, Vol. 15, 100-104

Bach J.R. (1995). Comprehensive rehabilitation of the severely disabled ventilator-assisted individual. *Monaldi Arch Chest Dis*, 48, 331-345.

Baxt W.G.(1992). Analysis of the clinical variables driving decision in anartificial neural network trained to identify the presence of myocardial infarction. *Ann Emerg* Med, 21, 1439-1444.

Boon M.E. & Kok L.P. (1995). Neural network processing can provide means to catch errors that slip through human screening of pap smears. *Diagn Cytopathol*, 9, 411-416.

Brooks SL.(1995). Computed tomography, *Dent Clin North Am*, 37, 575-590.

Buchanan B.G. & Shortliffe E.H. (1997. Rule Based expert systems : *The MYCIN experiments of the stanford Heuristic Progarmming Project*. Reading, Mass : Addison-Wesley.

Buning M.E .& Hanzlik J.R. (1995). Adaptive computer use for a person with visual impairment. *Am J Occup Ther*, 47, 998-1008.

Burke H.B. (1996). Artificial neural networks for cancer research : outcome prediction. *Semin Surg Oncol*, 10, 73-79.

Caillat S., Garchon H.J., Costantino F. & al. (1995). Automation of large scale HLA oligotyping using a robotic workstation. *Biotechniques*, 15, 526-528.

Cannavo S, De Natale R, Curto L & al. (1992). Effectiveness of computer assisted perimetry in the follow-up of patients with pituitary microadenoma responsive to medical treatment, *Clin Endocrinol*, 37, 157-161.

Cappini G, Poli R, Rucci M, & al. (1992), A neural network architecture for understanding discrete three dimensional scenes in medical imaging. *Comput Biomed Res*, 25; 569-585.

Cendrowska J. & Bramer M.A. (1984). A rational reconstruction of the MYCIN consultation system. *Int J Man-Machine Studies*, 20, 229-317.

Charniak E & McDermott D. (1989). *Introduction to artificial intelli-*

gence., Addison Wesley Publishing .

Chawanya T, Aoyagi T, Nishikawa I & Okuda K. *(1995).* A model for feature linking via collective oscillations in the primary visual cortex. *Biol Cybern,* 68, 483-490.

Clancey W.J. & Letsinger R. (1991) . NEOMYCIN : reconfiguring a rule based expert system for applications to teaching. In : *Proc IJCAI-81,* 2, 829-836.

Cohen IL, Sudhalter V, London D & al. (1995). A neural network approach to the classification of autism. *J Autism Dev Disord,* 23, 443-466.

Edenbrandt L., Devine B.& Macfarlane P.W. *(1995).* Classification of electrocardiographic ST-T segments - human expert vs artificial neural network. *Eur Heart J,* 14, 464-468.

Elstein A.S., Shulman L.A. & Sprafka S.A. (1992). *Medical problem solving : an anlysis of clinical reasoning.* Cambridge, Mass : Harvard Univ Press.

Fischer D, Wolfson, H & Nussinov R, (1995). Spatial sequences-ordering dependent structural comparison of alpha/beta pro-teins : evolutionary implications. *J Biomol Struc Dyn,* 11, 367-380.

Ganger M., Begin E. & Hurteau R. (1996). Robotic interactive laparoscopic cholecystectomy, *Lancet,* 596-597.

Hasan J., Hirvonen K., Varri A. et al. (1995). Validation of computer analysed polygraphic patterns during drowsiness and sleep on-set. *Electroencephalogr Clin Neurophysiol,* 87, 117-127.

Heiden W., Moeckel G. & Brickmann J. (1995). A new approach to analysis and display of local lipophilicity / hydrophilicity mapped on molecular surfaces. *J Comput Aided Mol Des,* 7, 503-514.

Hinton G.E. (1992). How neural networks learn from experience. *Sci Am,* 267, 144-151.

Kaplan SJ. (1994), The industrialization of artificial intelligence : from by line to bottom-line. *AI magazine;* 34 : 345-351.

Kappen H.J. & Neijt J.P. (1995). Advanced ovarian cancer. Neural network analysis to predict treatment outcome. *Ann Oncol,* 4, 31-34.

Kulikowski C.A. & Weiss S.M. (1992). Representation of expert knowledge for consultation : the CASNET and EXPERT projects. In : Szolovits P, ed. *Artificial intelligence in medicine.* Boulder, Colorado : Westview Press, 21-56.

La Fianza, A., Giorgetti S., Marelli P. & Campani R. (1995). Vocal recognition and oral radiology, *Radil Med*, 86, 432-435

Landi,s N.T. (1993). Pharmacies gain staff time as new "employee" lends a hand. Am *J Hosp Pharm*, 50 : 2236-2242.

Martin, LM. (1995). Computer assisted interpretation of resolution visual fields from patients with chiasmal and retrochiasmal lesions. *Ophtalmologica*, 207 : 148-154

Matesen, F.A, Garbini J.L. (1993). Robotic assistance inorthopaedic surgery. A proof of principle using distal femoral arthroplasty. *Clin Orthop*, 296 : 178-186.

Miller, A.S., Blott B.H., & Hames T.K. (1992). Review of neural network applications in medical imaging and signal processing, *Med Biol Eng Comput*, 30,449-464.

Miller, R.A., Pople H.E. & Myers J.D. (1992). INTERNIST-1, an experimental compute based diagnostic consultant for general internal medicine, *N Engl J Med*, 307, 468-476.

Miyashita Y, Date A & Okuno H. (1995), Configurational encoding of complex visual forms by single neurons of monkey temporal cortex, *Neuropsychologia*, 31, 1119-1131.

Modai I. (1993), Clinical decisions for psychiatric inpatients and their evaluation by a trained neural network, *Methods Inf Med* , 32; 396-399.

Mrosek B., Grunupp A., Keppel E. et al. (1995). Computer assisted speech recognition and display of x-ray findings, *Rofo Fortschr Geb Rontgenstr Neuen Bildgeb Verfahr*, 5 : 481-483.

Ng W.S., Davies B.L., Timoney A.G., et al. (1993). The use of ultrasound inautomated prostatectomy. *Med Biol Eng Comput*, 31, 349-354.

Nilsson J. (1990). *Principles of artificial intelligence*, Morgan Kaufmann Publishers Inc.

Pauker, S.G. & Szolovits P. (1997). Analysing and simulating taking the history of the present illness : concept formation. In : Schneider W, Hein A-LS, eds. *Computational linguistics in medicine*. Amsterdam: North Holland.

Pauker, S.G., Gorry G.A. & Kassirer J.P. (1996). Towards the simulation of clinical cognition : taking a present illness by computer. *Am J Med*, 60; 981-986.

Pople, H.E. (1985). Evolution of an expert system : from internist to caduceus. In : De Lotto I, Stefanelli M, eds. *Artificial Intelligence in medicine*; Survey lectures, 1-30.

Powers, R.K. (1995). A variable threshold motoneuron that incorporates time and voltage-dependent potassium and calcium conductances, *J Neurophysiol*; 70; 246-262.

Regia, J.A. (1993). Neural computation in medicine. *Artif Intell Med*, 5, 143-157.

Robertson, D.D. (1996). Distal loss of femoral bone following total knee arthroplasty. Measurement with visual and computer processing of roentgenograms and dual-energy x-ray absorptiometry. *J Bone Joint Surg Am*, 76, 66-76.

Ruppin E., Hermann M. & Usher M. (1995). A neural model of the dynamic activation of memory, *Biol Cyber*, 68,455-463.

Sompolinsky, H. & Seung H.S. (1993). Simple models for reading neuronal population codes, *Proc Natl Acad Sci USA*, 90,10749-10753.

Tadano, J. (1995). Robot handling system and conveying system of hospital laboratory, *Rinsho Byori*, 95 : 23-31.

Taylor, B., Cupo M.E. & Sheredos S.J. (1993).Workstation robotics : a pilot study of a Desktop Vocational Assistant Robot, *Am J Occup ther*, 47, 1009-1013.

Tu, J.V. & Guerriere M.R. (1995). Use of neural network as a predictive instrument for length of stay in the intensive care unit following cardiac surgery. *Comput Biomed Res*, 26, 220-229.

Turban, E. (1995). *Decision support and expert systems*, Macmillan Publishing Comp.

Turban E. (1994), *Expert systems and applied artificial intelligence*, Macmillan Publishing Comp.

Vyborny C.J. & Giger M.L. (1996). Computer vision and artificial intelligence in mammography, *Am J Roentgenol*, 162, 699-708.

Weiss S.M., Kern, K.B. & Kulikowski, C. (1992). *A guide to the use of the EXPERT consultation system*, Brunswick, New Jersey : Rutgers Univ, Report CBM-TR-94.

Wickham, J.E. (1994). Minimally invasive surgery. Future developments, *BMJ*, 308, 193-196.

Wilson, R.K. (1995). High throughput purification of M13 templates for DNA sequencing. *Biotechniques*, 15, 414-416.

Wolberg W.H., Street W.N. & Mangasarian O.L. (1995). Breast cytology with digital image analysis. *Anal Quant Cytol Histol*, 15, 396-404.

Zipser D., Kehoe B., Littlewort G., et al. (1993). A spiking network model of short term active memory, *J Neurosci*, 13, 3406-3420.

Chapter VII

An Intelligent Data Mining System to Detect Healthcare Fraud

Guisseppi A. Forgionne
Aryya Gangopadhyay
Monica Adya
University of Maryland Baltimore County, USA

INTRODUCTION

There are various forms of fraud in the health care industry. This fraud has a substantial financial impact on the cost of providing healthcare. Money wasted on fraud will be unavailable for the diagnosis and treatment of legitimate illnesses. The rising costs of and the potential adverse affects on quality healthcare have encouraged organizations to institute measures for detecting fraud and intercepting erroneous payments.

Current fraud detection approaches are largely reactive in nature. Fraud occurs, and various schemes are used to detect this fraud afterwards. Corrective action then is instituted to alleviate the consequences. This chapter presents a proactive approach to detection based on artificial intelligence methodology. In particular, we propose the use of data mining and classification rules to determine the existence or non-existence of fraud patterns in the available data.

The chapter begins with an overview of the types of healthcare fraud. Next, there is a brief discussion of issues with the current fraud detection approaches. The chapter then develops information technology based approaches and illustrates how these technologies can improve current practice. Finally, there is a summary of the major findings and the implications for healthcare practice.

BACKGROUND

Fraud in healthcare transactions refers to knowingly and willfully offering, paying, soliciting, or receiving remuneration to induce business that healthcare programs will reimburse. Healthcare fraud can result from internal corruption, bogus claims, unnecessary health care treatments, and unwarranted solicitation. As in any commercial enterprise, unscrupulous provider or payer employees can misappropriate healthcare payments for personal purposes. Providers can also issue claims for treatments that were never, or only partially, rendered. Corrupt healthcare providers also can induce patients to undergo unnecessary, or even unwanted, treatments so as to inflate charges to the payers. In addition, unethical providers can willfully solicit business from unprincipled, or unsuspecting, patients for the sole purpose of generating billable procedures and treatments.

According to a 1993 survey by the Health Insurance Association of America of private insurers' healthcare fraud investigations, the majority of healthcare fraud activity is associated with diagnosis (43%) and billing services (34%). In Medicare, the most common forms of fraud include billing for services not furnished, misrepresenting the diagnosis to justify payment, falsifying certificates of medical necessity, plans of treatment and medical records to justify payment, and soliciting, offering, or receiving a kickback (Health Care Financing Administration, 1999).

Early cases of healthcare fraud have applied to gross issues such as kickbacks, bribes, and other fairly transparent schemes. Increasingly, however, the Office of the Inspector General has demonstrated a willingness to pursue cases that are in the gray area and courts have tended to interpret antifraud statues more broadly so as to make criminal prosecution more likely (Steiner, 1993). For instance, waiving a patient's co-payment when billing third-party payers and not disclosing the practice to the insurance carrier has been deemed as fraud and resulted in prosecution (Tomes, 1993).

Fraud has a substantial financial impact on the cost of providing healthcare. Medicaid fraud, alone, costs over $30 billion each year in the United States (Korcok, 1997). According to CIGNA HealthCare and Insurance groups, the healthcare industry is losing an estimated $80 to $100 billion to fraudulent claims and false billing practices (CIGNA, 1999). Investigators have shown that fraud is found in all segments of the healthcare system, including medical practice, drugs, X-rays, and pathology tests, among others.

The timely detection and prevention of fraud will not only provide significant cost savings to insurance companies but will also reduce the rising cost of healthcare. Money wasted on fraud will be unavailable for the diagnosis and treatment of legitimate illnesses. In the process, research monies may be reduced and critical research may be delayed. Ineffective and cost inefficient treatments may continue. Administrative effort may be diverted to fraud detection instead of being concentrated on the effective management of healthcare practice. As a consequence, patient care may suffer and healthcare costs may continue to soar.

MAIN THRUST OF THE CHAPTER

There are several issues, controversies, and problems associated with fraud detection. An analysis of these issues recommends a solution based on artificial intelligence techniques.

Issues, Controversies, and Problems

In the past, claim fraud has been identified through complaints made, among others, by disgruntled healthcare competitors, beneficiaries and recipients, and present or former employees of providers. A significant volume of false claims, however, still go undetected. Consequently, fraud is still rampant in the healthcare system. The rising costs of, and the potential adverse effects on quality health care, have encouraged organizations to institute measures for detecting fraud and intercepting erroneous payments, especially through electronic means.

Due to the documentation typically required by payers, all forms of healthcare fraud will leave a paper, or electronic, trail that can serve as the basis for detection. However, the transactions useful for fraud detection will generally be buried in the documentation. Furthermore, these transactions may be from disparate sources and in diversified formats. Often, the needed transactions are also discarded as a normal part of transmitting claims from providers to payers.

Another major barrier to fraud detection is the reactive nature of the current approaches. For the most part, detection relies on: (a) complaints made by disgruntled interested parties, (b) random examinations by payers of provider submitted records, and (c) occasional detailed studies by public and private oversight agencies (Tomes 1993). Since such methods tend to be relatively narrow in scope, few fraud cases will be detected in this manner. Even in the identified cases, detection will be time consuming, costly, and difficult to correct.

Solutions and Recommendations

With the increasing number of healthcare transactions and persecution of situations with such uncertainty, it is possible to increase the chances of detecting fraud through the use of information technology. Such technology can be utilized to develop a proactive and effective healthcare fraud detection strategy based on data warehousing, data mining, artificial intelligence, and decision support systems.

Data needed to support the identification of fraud routinely flow, often electronically, between healthcare providers and payers as medical transactions. By filtering and focusing the transactions, warehousing the focused data, and creating tailor-made data marts for the appropriate recipients, requisite information can be made available for significant data mining analyses (Abraham and Roddick, 1998; Davidson, Henrickson, Johnson, Myers, and Wylie, 1999). Artificial intelligence then can be used to help providers and payers detect the underlying fraudulent patterns in the data and, with the aid of additional information technology, form effective proactive correction strategies (Burn-Thornton and Edenbrandt, 1998; Hornung, Deddens, and Roscoe, 1998; Makino, Suda, Ono, and Ibaraki, 1999).

Data Warehousing

Data warehousing involves the physical separation of day-to-day operational healthcare data from decision support systems. Benefits of data warehousing include clean and consistent organization-wide data, protection of transactional and operational systems from user's query and report requirements, and effective updating and maintenance of applications. The more significant purpose of the data warehouse is to support multidimensional analyses of both historical and current data.

A multidimensional model is developed using the MOLAP (multidimensional on-line analytical processing) design. Several data cubes are populated with historical and current data. An example of a three-dimensional data cube consists of patient demographics, time, and procedure code as the dimensions, and the payment as the measure. The actual analysis could require dimensionality reduction, such as a time-series analysis of payment records for patients that underwent a given treatment. In this case only two dimensions of the data cube are investigated. Such an analysis could be required to establish a historical pattern of the amount of payments made for a given medical procedure, sudden changes of which may cause an alarm for further investigations. Average values of payment amounts for medical procedures over a given data set can be used as a normative value to trigger any significant variations in current payment amounts. Other examples of multidimensional analyses include pivoting or cross tabulating measures against dimensions, dicing the cube to study a subpopulation of the data collected over a period of time, and rollup or drill down along dimensions to study any changes that might have taken place along individual dimensions.

Data Mining and Classification Rules

Data mining is an emerging technique that combines artificial intelligence (AI) algorithms and relational databases to discover patterns with or without the use of traditional statistical methods (Borok, 1997). It typically employs complex software algorithms to identify patterns in large databases and data warehouses. Data mining can facilitate information analysis using either a top-down or a bottom-up approach (Limb and Meggs, 1995). While the bottom-up approach analyzes the raw data in an attempt to discover the hidden trends and groups, top-down data mining tests a specific hypothesis.

Effective data mining relies on an effective and representative data warehouse. By definition, data mining is a pattern discovery process that relies on large volumes of data to infer meaningful patterns and relationships between data items. Once the data is "mined" from the warehouse and patterns are cataloged, the patterns themselves can be converted into a set of rules (Borok, 1997). These rules that explain healthcare behavior will be coded into a rule-base and be used for analyzing individual instances.

Classification rules deal with identifying a class of regularities in data (Adam, Dogramaci, Gangopadhyay and Yesha,1998; Ramakrishnan 1997). A classification rule is an expression $(l_1 \leq X_1 \leq U_1)$ $\ddot{Y}$ $(l_2 \leq X_2 \leq U_2) \wedge \ldots (l_k \leq X_k \leq U_k) \rightarrow (l_y \leq X \leq U_y)$, where $X_1 \ldots X_k$ are attributes used to predict the value of Y, and $l_1 \ldots l_k$, $U_1 \ldots U_k$ are the lower and upper bounds of the corresponding attribute values, respectively. As an example, in detecting healthcare fraud, a classification rule would be $X \rightarrow (Y \leq l_y)$ or $(U_y \leq Y)$, where X is a surgical procedure and (l_y, U_y) is the prescriptive range of values for the payments made (Y).

A classification rule is said to have a support s if the percentage of all cases satisfying the conditions specified in the rule equals or exceeds the support. In other words, s is the ratio to the total number of cases where both X and Y values are within the specified ranges. The confidence c of a classification rule is defined as the probability that, for all cases where the value of X falls within its specified range, the value of Y will also be within the range specified for Y. In other words, c is the ratio of cases where the values of X and Y are within their respective specified ranges, to the total number of cases where only the X values are within the specified range. Both support and confidence can be user or system specified as percentages or ratios.

If the support for a certain rule is low, it indicates that the number of cases is not large enough to make any conclusive inference. In that case, no further analysis is done with the current data set. If the support is large but the confidence is low, the rule is rejected. If both the support and confidence exceed the values specified by the user (or system) then the rule is accepted. Such a case would trigger a flag for a potential fraud and recommend further investigation, which is done by isolating the cases that triggered the flag.

Illustrative Example

Take the instance of determining physician charges for a surgical procedure. Charges for this procedure may vary somewhat by, among other things, physician, location of the practicing facility, and the regulations of the insurance provider. It is challenging, therefore, to identify an acceptable and representative range of charges using traditional statistical techniques. This requires understanding the physicians' practice procedures, determining the practice patterns implicit in the data, and possibly identifying practice patterns over the past few weeks.

Data mining can discover such patterns in the historical data. More importantly, it can uncover atypical patterns of practice within a group. For instance, mining on a large sample of nationwide data may identify that for a simple dental procedure, physicians charge a fee of $45.00 to $60.00 in the state of Maryland. If there is a sufficient number of cases in the data warehouse that support the correlation between the procedure and the range of charges, then the support and confidence in this rule will be high. Otherwise the rule will be rejected and will not be included in the rule-base. If the rule is accepted, a new case regarding this procedure can now be compared against the rule and can trigger a fraud alert if the charges deviate significantly from those specified in the rule.

In another instance, data mining may support the analysis and understanding of temporary conditions which may be incorrectly triggered as a fraud alert. Suppose the classification rules above indicate an increase in the incidence of emergency hospitalizations than in other regions around the area. This deviation can set up a trigger whereby further analysis may reveal the presence of a high-risk construction facility for the next two years. This factor will allow the healthcare providers to prepare for the situation both during and after the construction activity and possibly aid in the prevention of emergency situations at this facility. Similar analysis can be used for chronic conditions such as breast or lung cancer in specific regions.

FRAUD DETECTION SYSTEM

In the next few sections, we suggest the development of a decision support system to support the identification of fraud in healthcare transactions. The architecture for this system is proposed in Figure 1. As this figure shows, the system interactively processes inputs into the outputs desired by healthcare users.

Inputs

The fraud detection system has a data base that captures and stores historical, and industry standard, data on healthcare providers, claims, and payments. These data are extracted from the data warehouse that captures the relevant transactions from the providers to the payers, and vice versa.

Provider information includes the name, address, ID, and other demographics. Claims information includes the patient ID, procedure code, charge, billing dates, and other financial statistics. Payment information includes the patient and provider IDs, deductibles, co-payments, covered remuneration, and relevant payment dates.

There is also a model base that contains classification rules and artificial intelligence algorithms. The classification rules would establish lower and upper limits, supports, and confidence levels for each covered procedure from historical data and industry standards. These rules would be derived through the data mining tool, and the classification algorithm would determine the support and confidence of the classification rules.

Processing

The health official (health plan administrator, auditor, or other staff assistant) uses computer technology to perform the fraud detection analyses and evaluations. Computer hardware includes an IBM-compatible Pentium-based microcomputer with 16MB of RAM, a color graphics display, and a printer compatible with the microcomputer. Software includes the SAS information delivery system running through the Microsoft Windows operating system. This configuration was selected because it offered a more consistent, less time-consuming, less costly, and more flexible development and implementation environment than the available alternatives.

Users initiate the processing by pointing and clicking with the computer's mouse on screen-displayed objects. The system responds by automatically organizing the collected data, structuring (estimating and operationalizing) the classification rules, and simulating fraud performance. Results are displayed on the preprogrammed forms desired by health officials. Execution is realized in a completely interactive manner that makes the processing relatively transparent to the user.

As indicated by the top feedback loop in Figure 1, organized data, structured classification rules, and fraud performance reports created during the system's analyses and evaluations can be captured and stored as inputs for future processing. These captured inputs are stored as additional or revised fields and records, thereby updating the data and model bases dynamically.

Figure 1: Fraud Detection Conceptual System Architecture

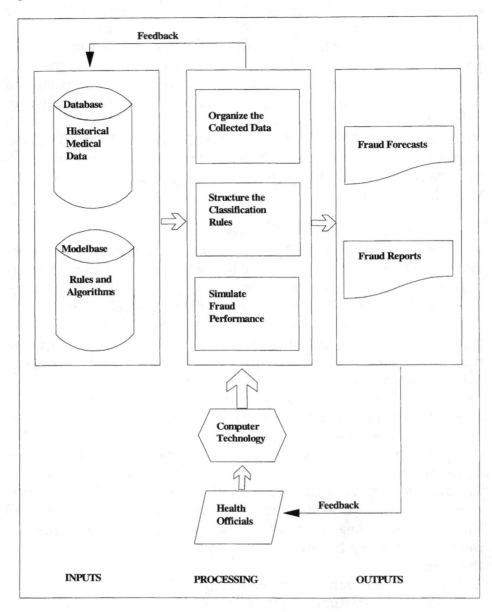

The user executes the functions with mouse-controlled point-and-click operations on attractive visual displays that make the computer processing virtually invisible (transparent) to the user.

Outputs

The above procedures generate visual displays of the outputs desired by health officials. Outputs include fraud forecasts and reports. These reports are in the form of tables and graphs. Each table displays the forecasted payment value relative to its lower and upper limits for a specified medical procedure. The corresponding graph highlights deviations outside the limits and allows the user to drill down to the supporting detail (which includes the provider, any extenuating circumstances, and other relevant information). The user has the option of printing or saving the reports.

As indicated by the bottom feedback loop in Figure 1, the user can utilize the outputs to guide further processing before exiting the system. Typically, the feedback will involve sensitivity analyses in which the user modifies support and confidence levels, upper and lower limits, or other pertinent factors and observes the effects on fraud performance.

System Session

There is a graphic icon on the Windows desktop. By double clicking this icon, the user accesses the fraud detection system. Once in the system, the user performs the fraud detection analyses and evaluations by navigating with point-and-click operations through the displays overviewed in Figure 2.

Figure 2: Display Relationships

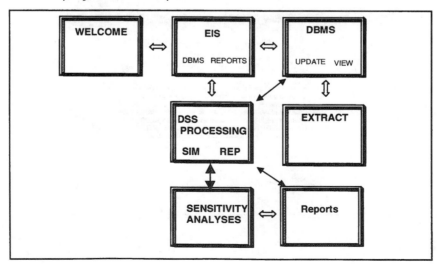

The Welcome display (shown in Figure 3) enables the user to access an embedded executive information system (EIS) shown in Figure 4. Once in the EIS, the user can interactively access the data warehouse, by selecting the database management system (DBMS) button, or go directly to DSS reports by selecting the REPORTS button. Selecting the DBMS button will enable the user to UPDATE the data warehouse and VIEW the contents of the existing or updated warehouse.

In the DBMS, the user can UPDATE the data warehouse and VIEW the contents of the existing or updated warehouse, as shown in

Figure 3: Welcome Screen

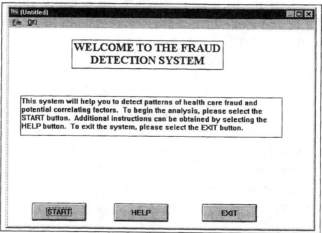

Figure 4: EIS Screen

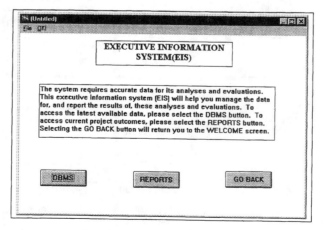

Figure 5. Selecting the UPDATE button will place the user in the EXTRACT screen shown in Figure 6. Once there, the user will interactively select the data source for the updating operation from the predefined list. The selection reads data from the specified source, reformats the data (if necessary), and updates the data warehouse values.

Selecting the VIEW button from the DBMS will access a display that prompts users for the desired information (shown in Figure 7). These selections will form the pertinent Structured Query Language (SQL) call to the data warehouse and generate the desired custom

Figure 5: Database Management System Screen

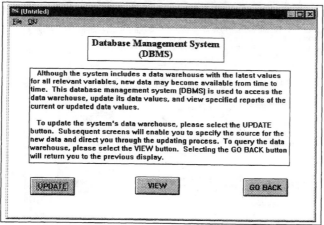

Figure 6: Extract Screen

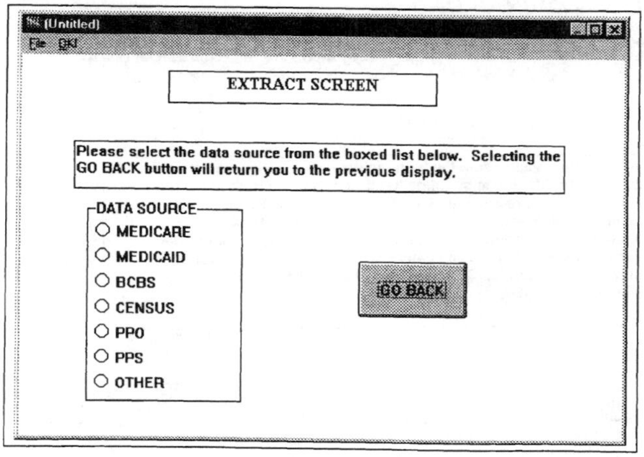

report.

Selecting the REPORTS button from the EIS display will run the fraud detection analysis with the updated or existing data and bring the user to the DSS PROCESSING screen shown in Figure 8. Once there, the user can simulate fraud performance by selecting the simulate (SIM) button. The decision support system will generate the required DSS database from the data warehouse, operationalize the appropriate models, and perform the needed analyses and evalua-

Figure 7: View Screen

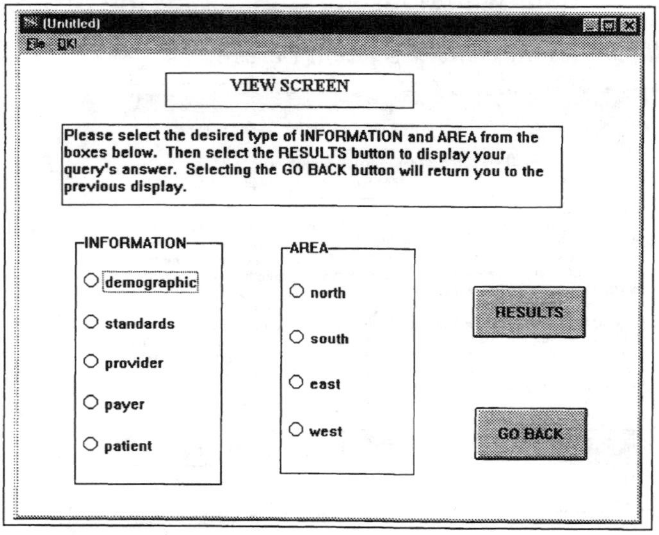

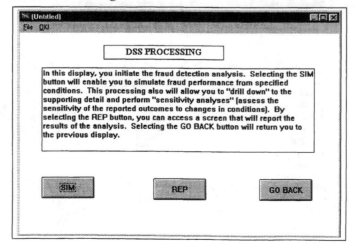

Figure 8: DSS Processing Screen

Figure 9: Reports Screen

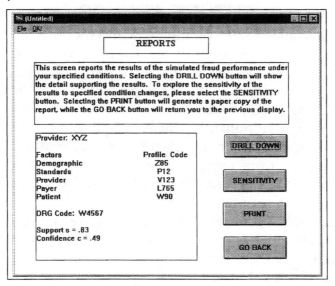

tions. It is here that data mining techniques will be used to identify new patterns in the updated databases. In deeper level screens, the user will be supported with features that allow the development of classification rules from patterns that hold consistently on data samples. These rules can then be used on incoming transactions to proactively identify fraudulent activities. A report (REP) button selection will display the results in the desired predefined format on the Reports screen (shown in Figure 9).

From the output screen, the user can perform sensitivity analyses on the results. By making the desired selection from the predefined "What If" list, the user can experiment with changes in: (a) provider characteristics, (b) key local factors, (c) patient demographics, and (d) financing alternatives. Results from the what-if analyses are displayed on the SENSITIVITY ANALYSES screen. Such experimentation can continue in sequence, or the user can generate an entirely new experiment.

Acting as an electronic counselor, the decision support system sequentially guides the user through an effective fraud detection analysis and evaluation. System operations, which are performed in an intuitive, timely (typical five-minute-session) and error-free fashion, liberate the user to focus on the creative aspects of fraud detection and correction.

FUTURE TRENDS

Web-based electronic commerce is an emerging trend that can benefit the healthcare community and the nation in a variety of ways. Such commerce enables the health care organization to be proactive rather than reactive. Transactions can be captured as they are generated, thereby allowing healthcare organizations to compare actual and expected patient outcomes. Such comparisons can help predict, among other things: (1) patient problems, (2) required healthcare interventions, (3) time required for implementation of healthcare services, (4) accessibility of healthcare services, (5) quality of healthcare services, and (6) cost of healthcare services.

The fraud detection system is conceived as a Web-based technology. A Web site will be established to collect the pertinent data from the various sources. Geographic data would be obtained from state and local government base map files, U.S. Postal Service ZIP Code files, U.S. Geological Survey hydrology data files, and U. S. Bureau of the Census TIGER files. General population characteristics would be obtained by census blocks from the U.S. Bureau of the Census, while health-related demographic data would be acquired from the U.S. Health Care Financing Administration and the National Health and Nutrition Examination Surveys. Health outcome and care data would be obtained from state-specific public health data files. Environmental data would be acquired from state and federal survey data files on water quality, pollutant, toxic waste, ambient air and source emission, air quality, radiation, powerline, and chemical usage and waste generation.

Utilizing the electronic commerce concept, data suppliers will access the system's Web site and select appropriate screen icons (Gerull and Wientzen, 1997). These selections will automatically obtain the data from the supply source and transfer the elements to a data warehouse (Tsvetovatyy, Gini, and Wiecckowski, 1997).

The system's EIS will extract the pertinent data, capture the extractions in user-oriented data marts, and make the marted data available for ad hoc queries by users. Ad hoc queries can be made at the users' sites in an easy-to-use, convenient, and interactive manner, utilizing the Web-based fraud detection system. Results will be displayed in formats anticipated by the requesting parties.

In effect, then, the proposed system provides a vehicle to utilize the emerging Web-based electronic commerce for proactive fraud detection and correction. Without the system, fraud detection involves a very complex process that requires extensive training for provider and payer analysts. By decreasing the volume of documentation, by simplifying the educational process, and by simplifying and automating much of the detection process, the proposed system can be expected to save the medical community millions of dollars per year in fraud detection and correction costs.

With the embedded EIS, an analyst can interactively conduct the initial phase of fraud detection at a computer terminal in a matter of minutes at a nominal expense. Next, the EIS can be used to access pertinent data, mine patterns from the accessed data, and relate the pattern variables with other correlates. The DSS then can be used to develop an explanatory model and use the model to simulate fraud performance under selected conditions. The fraud detection system can be developed and implemented for a small fraction of the potential cost savings.

From a diagnosis perspective, the manual search for fraud detection patterns is a tedious process that often results in inaccurate, incomplete, and redundant data. Such data problems can leave fraud inadequately detected and corrected. With the proposed system, the user identifies all data relevant to the fraud detection process, and the system provides a mechanism that facilitates data entry while reducing errors and eliminating redundant inputs. Reports from the system also offer focused guidance that can be used to help the user perform fraud searches, detections, and corrections.

Challenges

Realizing the strategic potential will present significant challenges to the traditional healthcare organization. Tasks, events, and processes must be redesigned and reengineered to accommodate the concurrent electronic commerce. Clinicians and administrators must be convinced that the electronic commerce will be personally as well as organizationally beneficial, and they must agree to participate in the effort. Finally, the organizational changes will compel substantial informational technology support.

The organization can have several stand-alone systems to provide the decision analyses and evaluations (Tan, 1995; Tan and Sheps,

1998). Integrating the stand-alone functions, however, can enhance the quality and efficiency of the segmented support, create synergistic effects, and augment decision-making performance and value (Forgionne and Kohli, 1996).

When implemented fully, the innovation will alter the work design for, and supervision of, fraud detection and correction. Requisite operations and computations will be simplified, automated, and made error-free. Training requirements will be reduced to a minimum. Processing efficiency will be dramatically increased. User-inspired creative fraud detection experimentation will be facilitated and nurtured. Management learning will be promoted. Knowledge capture will be expedited.

In short, the fraud detection system's usage would substantially reshape the organizational culture. Faced with significant time pressures and limited staff, healthcare leadership may be reluctant to take on this burden at the present time. In addition, public health officials have developed and cultivated strong and enduring relationships with practitioners and vendors. These practitioners and vendors also have important contacts and allies within the government agencies that oversee healthcare programs. For these reasons, it may be politically wise for public health officials to preserve these practitioner and vendor relationships.

Future Research Opportunities

There are a number of future research opportunities presented by the fraud detection system. To ensure that the information system accurately replicates the inputs, the final version of the system should be tested against Web-collected data from existing institutions. In the testing, warehoused data should be compared against actual values. Statistical tests should be conducted on the estimated models. There should be evaluations of user satisfaction with: (a) the speed, relevance, and quality of ad hoc query results; (b) the system interface; (c) model appropriateness; and (d) the quality of the system explanation. Simulations should be statistically tested for accuracy, and confidence intervals should be established for the results. Tests should also be conducted on the system's ability to improve the decision-making maturity of the user.

Enhancements can be made to the fraud detection architecture. Machine learning techniques can be developed to improve the intelligent modeling, database management, and user interface operations of the system. Communication links can be created to more effectively disseminate system results to affected parties.

The fraud detection system concept can also be adapted for a variety of adjunct healthcare applications. Similar systems can be applied to the diagnosis and treatment of cancer, mental disorders, infectious diseases, and additional illnesses. Effectiveness studies can be done to measure the economic, management, and health impacts of the additional applications.

CONCLUSIONS

The fraud detection system presented in this paper is a combination of data warehousing, data mining, artificial intelligence, and decision support system technology. This system offers the healthcare official a tool that will support a proactive strategy of health care fraud detection. The system's use can reduce the time and cost needed to detect healthcare fraud, and the system can substantially lower the public and private expenses associated with such fraud.

The fraud detection system delivers the information and knowledge needed to support fraud detection in a comprehensive, integrated, and continuous fashion. The comprehensive, integrated, and continuous support from the system should yield more decision value than the non-synthesized and partial support offered by any single autonomous system. Improvements should be observed in both the outcomes from, and the process of, strategic claims and other electronic commerce decision making (Lederer, Merchandani, and Sims, 1997). Outcome improvements can include advancements in the level of the users' decision-making maturity and gains in organization performance (Whinston, Stahl, and Choi, 1997). Process improvements can involve enhancements in the users' ability to perform the phases and steps of decision making.

To achieve the potential benefits, healthcare officials will have to meet significant challenges. First, a data warehouse must be established to capture the relevant transactions. In particular, there must be continuous user-involvement including careful upfront examination of business requirements and identification of quality and standards. The warehouse must be iteratively developed to deliver increasing value to the organization. Second, to support effective data mining, data marts must be formed to filter and focus the data for fraud detection. A strategy must be formulated for developing the tool. Once again, because of their domain knowledge, users must play a central role in such development. Thirdly, appropriate data mining techniques should be made available to the user and more importantly, validation routines will need to be built into the system to support effective validation of data mining outcomes. Finally, users must be convinced about the efficacy of the fraud detection system and trained in the use of the proactive technology.

Regardless of the proposed system's legacy, the application offers useful lessons for Web-based healthcare decision technology systems' development and management. The system is effectively delivering to the user, in a virtual manner, embedded statistical, medical, and information systems expertise specifically focused on the health care problem. Any single human technical specialist typically will not: (a) be proficient with, or even aware of, all pertinent tools, or (b) possess sufficient domain knowledge to fully understand the medical situation, propose trials, or interpret outcomes. While practitioners will have the domain knowledge, they usually will not have the technical expertise to effectively develop and implement relevant technology.

The proposed effort suggests that system design, development, and implementation should be a team effort. In addition, the team should be composed of the affected practitioners, information system personnel, and technological specialists proficient with the tools needed to address the healthcare problem.

Fraud detection is inherently a semi-structured (or even ill structured) problem. When initially confronted with such situations, analysts have a partial understanding of the problem elements and relationships. Typically, their understanding evolves as they acquire more information, knowledge, and wisdom about the problem. The fraud detection system is designed to support such decision making.

Relying on the information center, or other traditional information system organization, to design and develop a Web-based fraud detection system will likely be ineffective. These types of organizations typically are staffed by personnel with general skills, limited technological expertise, and restricted problem-specific knowledge. Development and implementation will follow a prescribed pattern designed to provide standard solutions to relatively well-understood and well-structured problems.

A hybrid project-technology organization may work well for Web-based fraud detection system design, development, and implementation in a healthcare environment. The organization would be virtual rather than physical. A project team would be established and administered by the practicing healthcare professional. Team technology specialists would be drawn from within and outside the organization to match the expertise needed for the specific project. Telecommuting and distributed collaborative work would be allowed and possibly encouraged.

REFERENCES

Abraham, T., & Roddick, J. F. (1998). Opportunities for knowledge discovery in spatio-temporal information systems. *Australian Journal of Information Systems*, 5(2), 3-12.

Adam, N. R., Dogramaci, O., Gangopadhyay, A., & Yesha Y. (1998). *Electronic Commerce: Technical, Business and Legal Issues.* New Jersey: Prentice-Hall.

Adam, N. R. & Gangopadhyay, A. (1997). *Database Issues in Geographic Information Systems.* Boston/Dordrecht/London, Kluwer Academic Publishers.

Borok, L. S. (1997). Data mining: Sophisticated forms of managed care modeling through artificial intelligence. *Journal of Health Care Finance.* 23(3), 20-36.

Burn-Thornton, K. E., & Edenbrandt, L. (1998). Myrocardial infarction—Pinpointing the key indicators in the 12-lead ECG using data mining. *Computers and Biomedical Research.* 31(4), 293-303.

Chen, R. (1996). Exploratory analysis as a sequel to suspected increased rate of cancer in a small residential or workplace community. *Statistics in Medicine,*15, 807-816.

CIGNA (1999). CIGNA HealthCare and Insurance Groups Web-site at http://www.insurance.ibm.com/insur/cigna.htm.

Davidson, G. S., Hendickson, B., Johnson, D. K., Meyers, C. E., & Wylie, B. N. (1999). Knowledge mining with VxInsight: Discovery through interaction. *Journal of Intelligent Information Systems: Integrating Artificial Intelligence and Database Technologies.* 11(3), 259-285.

Fischer, M. M. and Nijkamp, P (eds.) (1993). *Geographic Information Systems, Spatial Modeling, and Policy Evaluation.* New York: Springer-

Verlag.

Forgionne, G. A. and Kohli, R. (1996). HMSS: A management support system for concurrent hospital decision making. *Decision Support Systems*. 16, 209-223.

Grimson, R. C. and Oden, N. (1996). Disease clusters in structured environments. *Statistics in Medicine* 15, 851-871.

Geographic Information System for the Long Island Breast Cancer Study Project (LIBCSP). National Cancer Institute's Electronic RFP Number NO2-PC-85074-39. Bethesda: National Cancer Institute, 1998.

Gerull, D. B. and Wientzen, R. (1997). Electronic commerce: The future of image delivery. *International Journal of Geographical Information Systems*. 7(7) 38-51.

Heath Care Financing Administration. (1999). Medicare fraud Website at http://www.hcfa.gov/medicare/fraud.

Hornung, R. W., Deddens, J. A., & Roscoe, R. J. (1998). Modifiers of lung cancer risk in uranium miners from the Colorado Plateau. *Health Physics*. 74(1), 12-21.

Huxhold, W. E. (1991). *An Introduction to Urban Geographic Information Systems*. Oxford: Oxford University Press.

Kalakota, R. and Whinston, A. B. (1997). *Electronic Commerce: A Manager's Guide*. Reading, Massachusetts: Addison-Wesley.

Keegan, A. J. and Baldwin, B. (1992). EIS: A better way to view hospital trends. *Healthcare Financial Management*, 46(11), 58-64.

Korcok, M. (1997). Medicare, Medicaid fraud: A billion-dollar art form in the US. *Canadian Medical Association Journal*. 156 (8), 1195-1197.

Laden, F., Spiegelman, D., and Neas, L. M. (1997). Geographic variation in breast cancer incidence rates in a cohort of U. S. women. *Journal of the National Cancer Institute* 89, 1373-1378.

Lederer, A. L., Merchandani, D. F., and Sims, K. (1997). The link between information strategy and electronic commerce. *Journal of Organizational Computing and Electronic Commerce*. 7(1), 17-25.

Limb, P.R., and Meggs, G. J. (1995). Data mining -tools and techniques. *British Telecom Technology Journal*. 12(4), 32-41.

Makino, K., Suda, T., Ono, H., & Ibaraki, T. (1999). Data analysis by positive decision trees. *IEICE Transactions on Information and Systems*. E82-D(1), 76-88.

Oden, N., Jacquez, G., and Grimson, R. (1996). Realistic power simulations compare point- and area-based disease cluster tests. *Statis-*

tics in Medicine 15, 783-806.

Ramakrishnan, R. (1997). *Database Management Systems.* Boston: McGraw-Hill.

Regional Variation in Breast Cancer Rates in the U. S. – NIH. National Cancer Institute's Electronic RFA Number CA-98-017. Bethesda: National Cancer Institute, 1998.

Robbins, A. S., Brescianini, S., and Kelsey, J. L. (1997). Regional differences in known risk factors and the higher incidence of breast cancer in San Francisco. *Journal of the National Cancer Institute* 89, 960-965.

Steiner, J. E. (1993). Update: Fraud and abuse Stark laws. *Journal of Health and Hospitals.* 26, 274-275.

Sturgeon, S. R., Schairer, C., and Gail, M. (1995). Geographic variation in mortality rates from breast cancer among white women in the United States. *Journal of the National Cancer Institute* 87, 1846-1853.

Tan, J. K. H. (1995). *Health Management Information Systems.* Gaithersburg, Maryland: Aspen.

Tan, J. K.H., and Sheps, S (eds.)(1998). *Health Decision Support Systems.* Gaithersburg, Maryland: Aspen.

Tomes, J.P. (1993). *Healthcare Fraud, Waste, Abuse, and Safe Harbors: The Complete Legal Guide.* Chicago, Illinois: Probus Publishing Company.

Tsvetovatyy, N., Gini, M., and Wieckowski, Z. (1997). Magma: An agent-based virtual market for electronic commerce. *Applied Artificial Intelligence.* 11(6), 501-509.

Whinston, A. B., Stahl, D. O., and Choi, S. (1997). *The Economics of Electronic Commerce.* Indianapolis, Indiana: Macmillan Technical Publishing.

Workshop on Hormones, Hormone Metabolism, Environment, and Breast Cancer, New Orleans, Louisiana, September 28-29, 1995. *Monographs in Environmental Health Perspectives* supplement 1997, 105(3), 557-688.

Chapter VIII

Diabetes Mellitus — Evaluating the Diagnostic Probabilities

Adi Armoni
Tel-Aviv College of Management, Israel

The article examines the behavior of the human decision-maker. It surveys research in which about 90 physicians specializing in various fields and with different degrees of seniority participated. It tackles the question of whether it is possible to found the majority of the knowledge bases of the expert systems on the Bayesian theory. We will discuss the way of decision making conforming to the probabilities evaluated according to the Bayesian theory.

The logical conclusion, therefore, is that the development of a knowledge base for an expert system founded on probabilities calculated in accordance with the Bayesian theory must be carried out in a controlled manner and depend on the parameters mentioned above.

INTRODUCTION

In light of the many studies dealing with the representation of the knowledge in the knowledge bases of expert systems, and different methods of its operation, not enough attention has been paid to the difficulties involved in the elicitation of the knowledge required from the human expert. This applies particularly to the knowledge that is not strictly factual, but is mainly based on the experience and judgment of the human expert. From studies of this subject, it has become clear that the limitations of the decision-maker in dealing with uncertain information hurt the accuracy, quality, reliability, and consistency of his decisions (Armoni, 1995; Fischhoff 1982; Aase et al., 1996).

Until now the expert systems were based entirely on the evaluations of the human expert. They did not give further opportunity to test them by changing the acquisition direction and crossing the results received in contrast with the direct evaluations of the human expert (Fischoff and Beyth-Marom, 1983).

The classic model of development knowledge bases is based on the location of "THE" expert, identification of his expertise and elicitation of his knowledge.

DEFINITIONS

Probability Groups Evaluated

1) A priori probability—the prevalence of event K, hereby P(K), the evidence E hereby P(E), or the positive results in the testing X, hereby P(X).

2) Posterior diagnostic probability—the probability of the existence of the event K, when given evidence E, hereby P(K/E).

3) The conditional probabilities of evidence—the probability of existence of evidence E, given the occurrence of the event K, hereby P(E/K)

4) Posterior diagnostic probabilities of the test - the probability of the occurrence of event K when given positive results of test X. hereby P(K/X).

5) Conditional probability of the test—the probability of receiving positive results in test X, when given fact of occurrence of event K. hereby P(X/K).

Objective Probability

The values of the probability for which there is agreement in the professional literature (Thomas, Watkins and Ward, 1996; Martin and Hopper, 1998; Jensen et al., 1997; Jeffrey and Lisa, 1993; Ginsberg et al., 1985).

Consistency of Estimated Probabilities

The distance between the probabilities that were elicited directly and the same probabilities as they were calculated normatively ac-

Figure 1: The Concepts of Consistency and Accuracy in the Expert's Estimations

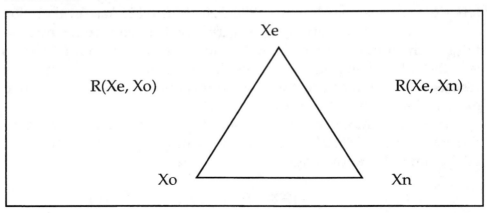

cording to the Bayesian theory.

Accuracy of the Estimated Probabilities

The distance between the group of probabilities that were estimated by an expert (directly or calculated normatively), and between their objective values.

In conclusion, the concepts of consistency and accuracy in the expert's estimations can be located through the following triangle (Armoni, 1995) :

Where:
Xe - Values of subjective probabilities as elicited from expert.
Xn - Values of probabilities as calculated normatively.
Xo - Objective values of probabilities.

The level of the consistency and the accuracy of the expert in his estimation of probabilities as expressed through the correlation :

R(Xe, Xn) - Degree of consistency of the expert .
R(Xe, Xo) - Degree of accuracy of the expert.
R is estimated by measures that will be described later in the study.

ASSESSMENT OF THE ACCURACY AND CONSISTENCY OF THE EXPERT'S ESTIMATIONS

Assessment of the Estimates Level of Consistency

1) Realization of the anomaly caused by lack of consistency by the expert (i.e. the proportion of calculated probabilities larger than 1).

2) The degree of fitness (if at all) between values of probability that were directly elicited, and those that were calculated normatively (i.e., the correlation coefficient) .

3) Quantitative concept for distance between the direct probabilities and the normatively calculated probabilities through average of absolute differences. In order to allow for the accurate estimation of differences between direct probabilities and normatively calculated ones, a confidence interval is determined for the value of Xdj (the direct evaluation of the expert).

Assessment of the Estimates Level of Accuracy

1) A quantitative measure of accuracy of the expert's estimations. Assessment of the distance between the expert's estimation and the objective values, through the average of absolute differences.

2) Assessment of the fitness between the expert's estimations and the objective values, as calculated by the correlation coefficient.

3) Sensitivity analysis of trends in the expert's estimates, whether he tends to overestimate, underestimate, or whether his estimations are accurate.

EMPIRICAL APPLICATION FROM THE FIELD OF MEDICAL DIAGNOSIS

General

Many expert systems have been developed for the field of medical diagnosis. As stated above, there is a fear within us questioning whether the probability values found in the knowledge bases of these systems express, accurately and consistently, the estimations of the human expert, who constituted the basis for the development of the system (Shortliffe 1997; Fryback 1997; Ben-Bassat et al., 1990). The disease that was chosen to represent the assumptions of the research is "Type 1 diabetes" (IDDM - Insulin Dependent Diabetis Melitus). This disease was chosen because of its complexity and complications on one hand, and its relatively high prevalence on the other hand.

Stages of the Empirical Experiment

The experiment involved four stages :

1) Elicitation of components of knowledge and construction of the questionnaire for the estimation of probabilities. The question-naire included 110 questions including a numeric scale (0-100) on which the estimating doctor was requested to indicate his estima-tion of the probability of events.

2) The initial sample included 13 internists and diabetologists. In response to their comments, the questionnaire was reduced to 75 questions and the wording was changed for part of the questions.

3) The use of the final version of the questionnaire for the population of doctors participating in the sample :

22 - endocrinologists / diabetologists

19 - internists

18 - family doctors

16 - pediatricians

03 - oncologists

08 - other doctors (orthopedists, surgeons, emergency, derma-tologists)

Overall, 86 doctors took part in the research. Each one of the doctors listed above completed the questionnaire together with a surveyor from the research staff.

4) An analysis of the research results and its recommendations for the method of eliciting information.

PRESENTATION AND ANALYSIS
OF THE RESEARCH RESULTS

1) According to all three measures of consistency defined in this study, there is a distinct preference (a=0.01) for endocrinologists in unconditional probability estimation and especially those re-lated to rare symptoms. Estimates of high levels of consistency were provided by pediatricians, especially concerning the diag-

nostic probabilities related to common symptoms. The internists and the doctors belonging to the group from various specialties, provided the estimates with the lowest level of consistency.

Suggested *explanation* for the findings described above can be attained from the fact that pediatricians first encounter the disease (juvenile diabetes), and as a result, have an advantage in the diagnosis of the disease and in the estimation of the diagnostic probabilities.

The endocrinologists on the other hand, specifically treat a population of diabetics, and are more exposed to cases with rare symptoms and complications related to the disease. Thus, they have an advantage in the estimation of the conditional probabilities.

2) A distinct preference in the consistency of the estimations, was discovered for the group of doctors with the maximal years of professional experience (20 years and more). It is clear from the results that as the number of years of professional experience of the estimating doctor increases, the consistency in his estimations increases, in accordance with the three measures of consistency that were described above.

3) The most accurate probability estimations for conditional probabilities groups with common symptoms related to Type 1 Diabetes were provided by pediatricians. The most accurate estimates for probabilities groups related to rare symptoms of Type 1 Diabetes were provided by endocrinologists. Note: the results mentioned above are distinct (alfa=0.01).

4) Contrary to the results received for the consistency of the estimations, the most accurate estimations were not necessarily provided by the doctors with the maximal years of professional experience. The most accurate estimations of a priori probabilities, and of conditional probabilities, especially those related to rare symptoms, were provided by doctors with professional experience of 11-20 years. The most accurate estimations for probabilities related to common symptoms were provided by doctors with the maximal years of professional experience (20

years and more).

Suggested explanation for those important findings might be credited by the "passion of research" mainly performed by a group of doctors with professional experience of 10-15 years. Thus, they have a relative advantage in estimating probabilities of rare symptoms.

On the other hand, the group of experienced doctors, exhibits a clear preference in their estimation of probabilities related to common symptoms, and this is of course due to their rich professional experience.

5) Positive correlation was found between experts that provided the most accurate estimates, and the groups who provided the most consistent estimates (alfa = 0.01). It is significantly clear that the experts who provided the most accurate estimates are the same ones who provided the most consistent ones.

THE CONTRIBUTION OF THE RESEARCH TO THE DEVELOPMENT OF KNOWLEDGE BASES FOR EXPERT SYSTEMS

1) The definition of measures and the development of techniques for the testing of internal consistency of the estimated probabilities. This technique is based on a numeric test of the estimated probabilities. The experiments that were done until now to test the consistency of the expert were based on the repeated questioning of the expert (regarding similar questions and different periods of time).

2) The definition of measures and development of techniques for the testing of accuracy of the expert's estimates. In this case, until now, a renowned expert was chosen, and the degree of accuracy in his estimates was not examined in any way.

3) Regarding the field of medical diagnosis, the study proves a positive correlation between the degree of consistency and the degree of accuracy of the expert.

The experts who are more accurate in their estimations are also the ones who show the most consistency. This finding is important especially in light of the fact that in part of the probabilities it is difficult (or even impossible) to locate the objective probabilities.

4) The study proves that differences in the degree of the consistency and accuracy of the knowledge elicited from the experts are dependent on professional characteristics and likewise, on professional expertise and number of years of experience. This contradicts the approach accepted today, according to which differences stem from personal characteristics only and are caused by difficulties which the individual encounters in his estimation of probabilities (Mark and Cookson, 1994; Shortliffe and Buchanan, 1975).

5) The findings from the empirical application of the methodology to the field of diagnostic medicine show that in contrast to the norm accepted today basing the development of knowledge bases of expert systems on the knowledge of a single expert.

It is necessary to build the knowledge base from the knowledge elicited from a number of experts from different professional expertise and with different numbers of years of professional experience. This exclusive recommendation comes from the "relative strength" (high degree of consistency and of accuracy) of each one of the experts in a different field of probabilities.

REFERENCES

Aase O., et al, (1996), "Decisions support by computer analysis of selected case history variables in the emergency room among patients with acute chest pain," *European-Heart-Journal*, Vol. 14, 433-440.

Armoni A., (1995), "Knowledge acquisition for medical diagnosis systems," *Knowledge-Based Systems*, Vol. 8, 223-226.

Ben-Bassat et al, (1990), "Sensitivity Analysis in Baysian Classification Models: Multiplicative Deviations" *IEEE Transactions on Pattern Analysis and Machine Intelligence*, PAMI-2(3), 261-266.

Fischhoff, B. (1982.), "Debasing in judgment under uncertainty : heuristics and biases," in Kahnman, D. Slovic, P. and Tversky, A., New York: Cambridge University Press.

Fischhoff, B. and Beyth-Marom, R. (1983), "Hypothesis evaluation from a bayesian perspective," *Psychological Review*, Vol. 90, 239-260.

Fryback, G. (1997), "Baye's theorem and conditional non independence of data in medical diagnosis," in *Computer assisted medical decision making Vol. 1*, Springer-Verlag, 183-195.

Ginsberg-Fellner M. et al, (1996), "Diabetes mellitus and auto immunity in patients with the Congenital Rubella syndrome," *Review of Infectious Diseases*, Vol.7 Supp.1, 170-176.

Jeffrey F, Lisa H. (1993) "Epidemiological approach to the etiology of type 1 diabetes mellitus and its complications," *The New England Journal of Medicine*, 317(22), 1390-1398 .

Jensen T, et al, (1997), "Coronary heart disease in young type 1 diabetic patients with and without diabetic nephropathy : Incidence and Risk factors," *Diabetologia*, 39(3), 144-148 .

Mark, D. Cookson, J. (1996), "The role of clinical judgment analysis in the development of medical expert systems," *Proceedings of the Second European Conference on Artificial Intelligence in Medicine*.

Martin F, and Hopper L, (1998), "The relationship of acute insulin sensitivity to the progression of vascular disease in long term Type 1 diabetes mellitus," *Diabetologia*, Vol 30, 149-153 .

Shortliffe, E.H. (1997), "Computer Based Medical Consultation : MYCIN," New York : Elsevier - North Holland, 175-210.

Shortliffe, E.H. and Buchanan, B.G. (1975), "A Model of Inexact Reasoning," *Medicine & Mathematical Biosciences*, Vol. 23, 351-379.

Thomas P, Watkins P, Ward J, (1996), "Diabetic Neuropathy. In Complications of Diabetes," 2nd edit. Kenn, H., and Jarrett, J Eds. London, Edward Arnold, 109-136.

Chapter IX

Telemedicine and the Information Highway

Bruno Lavi and Zeev Rotstein
Chaim Sheba Medical Center, Israel

Health systems broaden their importance in the midst of the ongoing international communications revolution. Health services are a natural candidate to become an integral part of the "information highway". Terms such as telemedicine, telehealth, teleradiology, and teledermatology have been integrated into technical and academic jargon and have become the object of research and organizational planning.

Telemedicine is the utilization of electronic technology to send medical data from one location to another. Supporting technology may be anything from a simple telephone, to complex communication satellite, and modern, videoconference equipment.

The term telemedicine is used to define the practice of medicine through communication technology. These two ancient words, medicine and communication, were first linked at the beginning of the 20th century, when ships used radio communication to receive medical assistance. It was only in the early 1960s, however, that link became truly significant. When we discuss communication from the technological aspect, we refer to the means permitting widespread transfer of information.

Improving access to information, minimizing cost, lowering professional isolation and improving quality of medical services are considered to be the main advantages offered by telemedicine.

The two central components affecting the success of telemedicine assimilation are the cost of service and the quality of service.

There is a clear and obvious correlation between technological development, in communications and other technological areas, such as image compression and adaptation, storage, and robotics, and advances in medical service in communication.

A basic and central element of telemedicine is the computer-based patient record. This subject has been widely discussed in the medical world, and is a central subject in the reform plans of American health systems.

Acceptance of telemedicine in the life of the individual and the health services organizations will demand a substantial change in clinical and organizational conceptions, and will result in a revolution in the existing health organizational structures, in treatment and diagnostic procedures, and in the health system policy as a whole.

BACKGROUND

Electronic communication continues to develop and evolve. Utilizing computer sources at distant locations is as popular today as was the use of typewriters 20 years ago. There are *online* commercial services such as CompuServe, automatic registers linked to banks in other countries, and companies with offices worldwide that routinely transfer information between distant sites.

The common denominator between all these sources is that they are all a part of an information channel *"network."* Communication over these networks enables computer stations to send and receive information without regard to distance.

There are few areas, if any, that will not benefit from taking advantage of the various information communication technologies. Utilization of information technology as a whole is particularly relevant to health and clinical systems. Ongoing advances in the various medical technologies, together with the desire to offer superior medical services to society, while giving consideration to cost and results, are just part of the reason for the widespread use of information technologies in health systems.

Factoring in the profusion of different services, the diversification and proliferation of insuring bodies, the growing self-awareness of personal health, and emerging medical advances then means that maintaining an active, effective communication channel between all the involved parties becomes complex and difficult. At the core of any attempt to deal with these difficulties is maintenance of an effective channel of open communication which includes collection and distribution of authenticated information between the various bodies involved.

Health systems broaden their relevance in the midst of the ongoing international communication revolution. Health services are a natural candidate to become an integral part of the *information highway*. Terms such as *telemedicine, telehealth, teleradiology, teledermatology,* and etc., have been integrated into technical and academic jargon and have become the object of research and organizational planning.

What Is Telemedicine?

Telemedicine is the utilization of electronic technology to transfer medical data from one location to another. Supportive technology can be anything from a simple telephone, to complex communication satellite, and modern, videoconference equipment.

Uses for telemedicine range from imaging (x-rays) to psychiatry. Telemedicine has already been used in the field of surgery, when a surgeon at one medical center was able to observe a medical procedure being executed at another medical center.

In Texas, telemedicine is utilized in the penal system, where incarcerated inmates are examined utilizing videoconference equipment. Physicians, who are experts in their field, can communicate via videoconference with patient inmates and make relevant observations and diagnoses.

In Oregon, a project is being set up to allow dermatological consultation through the transfer of a patient's dermatological images from the rural area where the patient lives to a dermatologist in Portland. This project will contribute to healthcare by saving financial expenditure on costly travel and allowing patients, even in the most peripheral areas, to receive quality dermatological consultation.

TELEMEDICINE—HISTORY AND ACCOMPLISHMENTS

Although it may appear that only during the last four to five years medicine has been assisted by communication technology, in fact, communication has been utilized for medical purposes since 1920, when radio communications connected the coastal medical stations with ships at sea to enable them to assist in medical problems.

More significant developments began 30 years ago with NASA's central role in medical communication (Bashshur & Lovett, 1977). NASA's efforts began in the early 1960s when man first conquered space. Physiological and medical data were transmitted between stations on earth to the astronauts either on board the space capsule or in pressurized spacesuits outside the space capsule. These early efforts and developments in satellite space communication encouraged the development of communication in medicine. The book by L. Rashid Bashshur, published in 1975 (Bashshur R.L. et al., 1975), mentioned approximately 15 projects in medical communication active at that time.

Some Pioneering *Telemedicine* Projects

STARPACH

Space technology applied to the Papago Native American Reservation in the state of Arizona (**STARPACH**) is one of the earliest experimental projects that supplied medical treatment to the Papago Native American Reservation in the state of Arizona. The project was initiated by NASA and operated between 1972-1975. The project was executed and evaluated by a team from Papago, Native American medical services, and the American Department of Health, Education and Welfare. The project's aim was to supply general medical services to the residents of the Papago Reservation. A truck manned by a team of two paramedics and equipped with ECG equipment, X-ray equipment, and a range of other equipment was hooked up to two local hospitals by two-way microwave radio set (Bashshur, 1980).

NEBRASKA MEDICAL CENTER

In 1955 the Nebraska State Psychiatric Clinic was among the first to have closed circuit television. Communication between the Norfolk

Government Hospital and the Nebraska State Psychiatric Clinic was made possible in 1964 through financing from a National Mental Health Institute research grant in the sum of $480,000. Doctors communicated educational and diagnostic information. In 1971 an additional line of communication was opened between the Nebraska State Medical Center and Veterans Hospital in Omaha, Nebraska, in an attempt to utilize this line for group therapy (Benschoter, 1971).

MASSACHUSETTS GENERAL HOSPITAL (MGH)

The Logan International Airport Health station was set up to supply medical services to airport employees, and preliminary and emergency healthcare to airplane passengers. Doctors from MGH supplied medical services to the health station patients via two-way circuit microwave television. The health station was manned by one nurse, 24 hours a day, and reinforced by an additional nurse when necessary. Patient diagnosis and treatment was decided upon by the nurse and carried out by MGH physicians. This included data taken by the physician, diagnosis of findings, x-ray evaluation, and microscope images. The nurse at the health station administered hands-on treatment when deemed necessary (Murphy and Bird, 1974).

ATS-6 ALASKA
Experiment in Physician Communication via Satellite

In 1971, 26 locations in Alaska were chosen by the National Library of Medicine, Lister Hill National Center for Biomedical Communication, to assess whether reliable communication could improve medical care in rural areas. Project evaluation was carried out by the University of Stanford Institute of Communication Research. Findings reported that satellite communication is applicable and productive in most medical services, with the exception of emergency services (lack of time for communication setup). It was demonstrated that among all emergency cases only 5-10% benefited from video communication. In the remainder of cases video communication was no more advantageous to the case than audio communication (Foote, 1977).

PRESENT DAY TELEMEDICINE

Communication and Medical Services

During the 1990s the concept of telemedicine penetrated the awareness of medical service suppliers, not as an experimental concept, but as an organizational and practical objective important in the supply of low cost, high quality, effective medical services.

The inherent potential of telemedicine is manifested mainly in the ability to supply medical data quickly, an ability necessary for making quick medical decisions by physicians in the relevant medical specialties and an ability independent of the physical location of the physician and patient.

Its primary use today is the transfer of clinical information and data between different locations: patient location to medical center, or medical center to medical center, and performing primary medical consultation between patients and specialist in distant locations. These applications will allow decentralization of medical services and be an important factor in affecting the patient's concept of medical needs, the quality of service, time required to receive service, and the patient's relationship with medical service suppliers.

Almost every branch of medicine and every medical subject is relevant and applicable to and through telemedicine, either wholly or in part, depending on the medical procedure and technological capabilities.

A NUMBER OF EXAMPLES OF MEDICAL SERVICES APPLICABLE TO TELEMEDICINE:

Teleradiology

Diagnostic Service Telecommunication. Video transfer of x-ray, CT, and MRI images between different locations for diagnostic consideration by videoconference allows radiological diagnosis on the same level as conventional diagnosis (Korsoff, 1995, Goldberg, 1994).

Telepathology

Consultation and Diagnosis Service through the transfer of microscopic finding images and videoconference. Improving technology (video technology, image compression technology, transfer time and communication capacity technology), while at the same time reducing cost, will contribute to developing medical pathology service in telecommunication.

Telepsychiatry
Psychiatric Analysis by Telecommunication. L. Baer has demonstrated in his research that the use of videoconference in analysis of patients diagnosed as suffering from Obsessive-Compulsive Disorder is an effective means of medical communication with distant areas, in no way affecting the quality of the service.

Psycho-Therapeutics
This branch of medical treatment has not, as yet, found a relevant treatment channel in telecommunication, at least not by any conventional concept (Kavanagh, 1995).

Home Nursing Services via Telecommunication
This is a rapidly developing branch of home nursing service. In the United States alone, it is expected that by the year 2030 more than 5 million people will enjoy this kind of service, and annual growth is expected to reach 12%.

Data such as blood pressure, pulse, ECG monitoring, follow up, and observation are at present already only a part of the nursing services data that can be transferred by telecommunication. It appears that telecommunication will become an integral part of nursing services in the future (Engstrom, 1996; Siwicki, 1996).

The aforementioned examples make up only a small part of the health services that can utilize telemedicine. In reality, any medical service which does not require hands-on treatment by the physician, or invasive treatment, can benefit from telemedicine, at the same time taking into consideration cost effectiveness, technology, information confidentiality, and other aspects governing the physician and medicine in general.

Human Aspects and Organization
Most researchers agree that the weak link in communication networks has been and remains the communication language between the user and the source of information. The keyboard, complex

computer directions, and the various ways of displaying data have blocked the path of many potential users. New approaches in communication techniques developed during recent years, such as the mouse, pull down menu, and touch screen, have somewhat improved and strengthened the connection between the computer and the computer user, making the computer more user friendly.

Further technological developments such as voice-recognition instructions, written instructions, and new computer languages may also help remove the barriers between some users and the computer technology.

The development of electronic communication and its penetration of the health systems impacts on management and management systems. Taking advantage of the relevant communication systems permits review, follow up, and better control at the management and decision-making level, by allowing easier access to updated information and data.

In the opinion of analyst Tom Peters (1988), successful organizations of the future will be comprised of more units and sub-units, each with more autonomy for defining both product and services, quality awareness, improved responses, and taking initiative. The central premise is that resources and the decision-making process should be in as close proximity as possible to the service staff and to the client. Modern communication technology will make information and knowledge available to individuals in remote areas.

Future world health organizations will, with the help of various forms of telecommunication, be able to transfer information sources and knowledge from their centers to their clients. Because telecommunication can transfer information more proximal to the client, organization management centers will be transformed from service centers into information centers.

Health organizations can exist in the communication network as *virtual organizations,* that combine with and connect between the hospitals, clinics and the individual patient.

Medical management personnel, physicians and researchers can communicate, via communication networks, for the purpose of transferring and exchanging information, completing monetary and managerial transactions, all within the framework of a decentralized, collaborative organization network.

Actually, the *virtual* health organization could, in the coming era, be the conduit for dispersion of medical services. Of course service users directly relate the efficacy of this technology to its compatibility, implementation, and acceptance. We can, of course, maintain that information technology is the major barrier to allowing telemedicine to becoming completely assimilated (and friendly). However, it is not perceived as such in ongoing projects and experiments (Moore, 1993).

Advantageous Use of Telemedicine

There is general consensus that telemedicine holds many advantages both for the information supplier and the user/customer. An evaluation by Moore of a number of projects in this field, carried out in 1993, presented the following advantages:

- **Improving Access to Information:** Telemedicine can supply medical services in areas where few medical services exist or where the existing services are not of good quality. It can supply small villages, peripheral communities, areas under siege of war, or areas where the ratio of physicians to population is low. Access to medical centers, and thus to physicians who are specialists in their field, via telecommunication permits faster and better quality medical service. Telemedicine can also shorten the time required for diagnosis. By conventional means this would first require a primary diagnosis by the family physician, followed by a request for medical confirmation from a medical center, a visit to the medical center, further evaluation and diagnosis, and then the patient would return to his family physician. Travel time would be shortened immeasurable by telecommunication. The family physician and physicians consulted through telemedicine are brought together through telecommunication. The diagnosis stage is shortened, and the need to travel back and forth for appointments is unnecessary.

- **Minimizing Cost:** Lowering and minimizing cost is accomplished by doing away with the costly and time-consuming need for the patients and/or the physicians to travel. Telemedicine can minimally reduce the need for patients to travel to physicians for consultation and evaluation, and likewise the need for physicians and specialists to travel to courses and seminars, thus allowing optimal exploitation of resources by preventing unnecessary duplication of services and manpower. Geographically conscience utilization of manpower and services—one physician can cover a vast geographical area.

- **Lowering Professional Isolation:** It is a proven fact that the collaboration of professional bodies via telemedicine, both at the diagnostic and evaluative stage, and during seminars and courses, lowers the level of professional isolation. Hartman and Moore (1992) found that 76% of the doctors, 92% of nurses, and 88% of paramedics who participated in telemedicine programs stated that their feeling of professional isolation was considerably lessened.

- **Improving Quality of Medical Services:** The challenge of successfully organizing a large number of medical personnel (attending physician, specialist, and family doctor) to deal with a specific medical problem, requires complex planning. Hartman and Moore (1992) describe the positive effect that the telemedicine conference has had on various medical organizations. This is expressed in the quality of service: a guarantee of quality, accurate information transferred between conferring medical organizations, recording telemedicine conferences enabling analysis of recorded information at a later date, exchange of ideas and information, and medical instruction.

  Unrestricted by geographic considerations, telemedicine facilitates instant organization of videoconferences. Telemedicine conferences not only shorten the diagnostic and evaluative processes, but also guarantee transfer of accurate and complete medical data between the various medical bodies.

Furtado (1982) described one application of telemedicine. In socio-therapeutic cases, the patient who is hospitalized at a distant location is able to have family "visits" via interactive television.

Telemedicine Cost, Investment and Returns

When calculating the cost of telemedicine, consideration must be given to the cost of software, hardware, ongoing expenditure on network services, upkeep, and manpower. Consideration must also be given to less tangible costs, such as time necessary for familiarization with new systems and adjustment time for service teams to new work locations.

In the past, the high cost of hardware was the primary obstacle to the implementation of telemedicine projects. Today hardware that formerly cost $100,000 can be attained for $15,000 and sometimes even less, thus rendering hardware cost much less of an obstacle.

Until now, very few financial analyses of telemedicine have been carried out, mainly because large medical insurance institutions would only occasionally acknowledge the insured party's expenses for this type of service. Some of the small number of evaluations done up until now are as follows:

- Utilizing telemedicine to connect between distant locations saves $1,000 per patient.
- More profit for medical service suppliers at less cost to patients/consumers.
- Return of initial investment two to three years into the project.

Medical insurance institution unwillingness to recognize these services, is a serious obstacle to the implementation of telemedicine (Williams & Moore, 1995).

One of the major cost elements of health service is manpower. This is an even more expensive element if the division of responsibility between the various parties (physicians, nurses, and paramedics) is not assigned effectively. Doctors, who are a much more expensive category of manpower, are doing many jobs that could be accomplished by nurses.

"We need to be asking what physicians are doing, and we need to be asking why nurses are not doing more" (Clinton 1993).

Cunningham, et al. (1978) investigated whether nurses could replace doctor's positions when implementing telemedicine. In pediatrics, the findings showed that diagnosis through closed circuit television allowed the doctor to effectively be replaced by a nurse 40% of the time.

Establishment and Duplication of Telemedicine

Most research in telemedicine has focused on the technological aspects, cost versus profit, areas of application and effectiveness, while the aspect of information assimilation (dissemination), problematic in every field, has been discussed very little and even then only in general.

At Memorial University Telemedicine Center (MUTEC), St John's, Newfoundland, Canada, telemedicine research projects have been developed continually over the past 30 years. Eight guidelines for the telemedicine assimilation process have been developed (M. House, 1991):

1. Use the cheapest and simplest technology applicable to existing needs.
2. Develop flexible systems, capable of adjusting and changing with new developments.
3. Involve all consumer groups on commencement of project.
4. Form support teams at the service sites.
5. Plan exact coordination between involved parties (organizational bodies and communication systems connected to the project).
6. Develop the cooperation of service consumers (of common interest).
7. Make plans to sustain continuation of the project after trial period.
8. Develop evaluation system (results, cost, effectiveness, etc.).

Generating Development of Telemedicine

As has happened in other areas, more has been invested in the technological development aspects of telemedicine than in making that technology available and applicable. Among the main factors influencing the general development of telemedicine are the following:

- **Cost - Profit Ratio**

  There is very little evidence for financial gain (what little there is relates to specific areas and branches).

- **Service Effectiveness**

  Different projects have demonstrated that by eliminating the need to travel to receive medical services or medical instruction, and the utilization of the *virtual* meeting between the parties involved, the effectiveness of telemedicine was proven beyond a doubt. The evidence gathered so far relates to relatively limited projects, whose effectiveness in a large community will, it follows, be commensurate to the defining perimeters.

- **Aspect of Medicine, Law, and Ethics**

  Many questions remain to be answered before the majority of telemedicine services (as opposed to experimental projects) can be implemented. Examples of these are questions related to responsibility for medical treatments via telemedicine, and application of medical license and law in different states and countries. The dilemma of securing information stored in the computer, which is also under discussion in other fields, is of supreme importance in medicine, both from the aspect of the possible consequences of changing medical data and the aspect of "confidentiality" of medical data. This dilemma will be discussed at length in another part of this work.

- **Guaranteeing the Quality of Medicine**
  There is no room for compromise regarding the quality of medical service. Even when technological advancement allows a total application of medical services via telemedicine, the subject of service quality will constantly need to be examined and evaluated. The absolute need to maintain a necessary level of quality must always come before any consideration of cost versus profit.

- **Defining Technical, Clinical, and Organizational Standards of the Service Suppliers**
  A necessary precondition to opening communication channels between the parties involved is technological suitability, agreement regarding clinical standards, and management methods.

- **Willingness of Potential Service Suppliers and Users**
  Another precondition to telecommunication application is potential service suppliers and consumer willingness to use the service.

As long as telemedicine is accepted by only a small percent of potential service suppliers and consumers, it cannot be activated on a large scale. Various groups, medical service suppliers, patients, insurers and subgroups exist, and in order for telemedicine to be activated, all of these groups and sub-groups must be prepared to participate (Drips, 1992).

Projects and Telemedicine Application (Appendix A)
If we consider a very general definition of telemedicine we can then assume that almost every medical organization makes use of some telemedicine services (telephone, fax, and computer). Use of the word telemedicine is becoming more widespread, as various forms of information technologies develop. Thus, when discussing various

projects and applications of telemedicine we mean those uses and applications where the technology produces added value. In the source, Telemedicine Information Exchange (http://tie.telemed.org), approximately 170 projects, in progress today worldwide, are mentioned. The majority of the projects are in the United States and Western Europe, but countries such as Greece, India, Thailand, and of course Israel, contribute as well. A look at the project summaries gives one the impression that the existence of telemedicine services in different countries is made possible by three things: the ability to invest in research and development (tens of thousand of dollars to millions of dollars), the physical size of the country (Australia, Canada, and the U.S.A., for example), and technological ability (Japan, Israel, U.S.A., for example).

The medical disciplines taking advantage of the telemedicine potential are many and various. Its use is particularly wide spread in areas where diagnosis is assisted by transfer of medical images (diagnostic imaging, skin diseases); test results data (cardiology, gynecology); or evaluation, treatment, and medical recommendations, as given by verbal and written instruction (psychiatry, medical instruction).

The following ongoing worldwide projects are the result of an existing need and illustrate the practical uses of telemedicine.

Australia

Australian National Antarctic Research Expeditions (ANAEW) Telemedicine Scheme, Polar Medicine Branch, Australian Antarctic Division, Channel Highway, Kingston, Tasmania 7050 Australia.

> **Contact:** Peter Sullivan MD, Medical Research Office: +61 02 323305
> (voice): + 61 02 323310 (fax): peter sul@antdiv.gov.au (e-mail): http://www.antdiv.gov.au/aad/pmed/med.html (WWW site)
> **System:** Store and forward
> **Applications:** Radiology and microscopic images
> **Technologies:** Nikon SLR Camera, Kodak DCS 200 CCD, Macintosh Powerbook, Mac Quadra Adobe Photoshop 3.0 imaging software, Tektronix Phaser II SDX color printer
> **Funding:** The Australian Antarctic Division is an agency of the Australian Federal Government.

A single doctor in each of four Australian Antarctic stations is supplying the complete range of medical services to the members of the various expeditions for one entire year. During most of the year, the transfer of a patient in need of medical services to medical centers is almost completely impossible. To minimize the station doctor's professional isolation, a system has been developed that enables contact with the relevant medical specialist and transfer of medical images to assist in diagnoses.

Israel

Shahal Medical Services Ltd., Ashdar Building, 90 Igal Alon St., Tel Aviv, 67891, Israel

Contact: Michael Benedek: 972-3-563 3888 (voice); 972-3-562 5727 (fax)

System: Interactive

Applications: Home health

Technologies: Tele-monitoring

Shahal Medical Services Ltd. was founded in 1987 to provide emergency and preventative medical service. These services are supplied via telephone communication with the consumer-patient and various evaluative medical equipment in the patient's home that transfer test results (ECG, BP, pulse, etc.) by telecommunication to the company's control center. On evaluation of the tests, and other medical considerations, a decision is made whether to send an ambulance team to the patient's home. In the patient's home the patient receives emergency medical treatment and/or the patient is transferred to the hospital. On arrival at the hospital, the patient has in his possession all the necessary up-to-date medical documentation regarding his condition.

Today, Shahal serves over 30,000 client patients. The company has expanded its services to the United States, Europe and Asia.

The State of Arkansas, U.S.A.

University of Arkansas for Medical Sciences (UAMS), 4301 Markham, Slot 599, Little Rock, AR 72205 U.S.A.

Contact: Ann Bailey Bynum, Ed.D., Program Assoc. Director, Area Health Education Centers: (501) 686-2590 (voice); (501) 686 2285 (fax); abbynum@life.uams.edu (e-mail): http.//uams.edu:80/ahec/tele 1.htm (WWW site).

System: Interactive

Applications: Trauma, emergency, cardiology, mental health, substance abuse, pediatric, obstetrics and gynecology, orthopedics, neurology, and education

Technologies: Four intra-campus sites linked by fiber optics, five area health education centers (AHECs) and seven affiliated rural hospitals liked by T1 lines.

Vendors: VTEL

Funding: University and state support, REA Grant - $ 1.5 million investment in network

This project was set up with the goal of improving accessibility of medical specialists to patients in rural areas. This is accomplished by utilizing an interactive television network that is part of State of Arkansas Network - STARNET, U.S.A.

State of California, U.S.A.

Tele-Psychiatry Program, P.O.B. 7549, Riverside CA. 92513-7549 U.S.A.

Contact: Richard Dorsey, M.D., Medical Director, Dept. of Mental Health, County of Riverside: (909) 358 4501 (voice); (909) 358 4513 (fax).

System: Interactive

Applications: Psychiatry

Technologies: Telephone consultation and video conferencing.

Vendors: PC/Codec, ISDN

Funding: Internal, $ 30,000

Telephone and videoconference technologies enable patients in remote areas to contact psychiatric services for consultation, diagnosis, treatment and other recommendations, or when consultation with a specialist is found necessary.

State of Florida, U.S.A.

Jackson Memorial Hospital/CHI/Telemedicine Project, Univ. of Miami, School of Medicine, Dept. of Dermatology, P.O.B. 016250 (R-250), Miami, Florida 33101, U.S.A.

System: Interactive

Applications: Dermatology

Technologies: AT&T ISDN line interfaces, Hitachi videoconferencing units; Microvix-S microscope video processor;

Panasonic video printer; Traga video capture boards; VideoMed image transmission software

Dermatologist specialists at Jackson Memorial Hospital (JMH) provide consultation services in diagnosing dermatological problems for patients at the Martin Luther King Jr. Clinica Campesina in Homestead, Florida via video conferencing. Between 10-15 patients receive consultation and diagnosis in each session. Physicians at JMH are able to adjust the cameras, enlarge the video image, save images, and access images from a certain file or print out, in color, the image they chose.

The aforementioned projects, and many similar ones, are only a sample of what we can expect telemedicine to develop into in the future. Their success, profitability, organizational and marketing value during coming years will set the standard for telemedicine application as part of the worldwide *information highway*.

Since the main sources of funding for these projects still come from research grants, and government research project funds, it is still too early to consider telemedicine either as a private or government venture, or as an integral part of ongoing national or international health services.

FINANCIAL ASPECTS

Telemedicine economics is today's focus and central subject in health systems research. Interest in this subject evolves mainly from a lack of experience in long-term activation of the telemedicine network.

As opposed to other fields, in reality, evaluation of health systems by cost-profit margin is not always based on monetary or numerical statistics alone. However, health systems managers around the world tend to attach growing importance to the financial aspects of health services. The goal is transforming health systems into genuine business enterprises, thus avoiding situations where, due to financial difficulties, the government is forced to pay out large sums of money to save the health system from bankruptcy (Kupat Holim in Israel, for example).

Today more than ever before, the application of new technologies in health service organization is seen from the financial aspect. Both the clinical value and the economic aspect are given equal consideration. Telemedicine, which is a collection of a wide variety of medical technologies, does not employ less decision makers (diagnosticians) than other medical technology services, if doing so is economically sound as well as clinically advisable.

Rapid technological development, along with a variety of complex evaluation indexes, accompanied by organizational and legal obligations, raises a wide variety of financial questions regarding the cost-profit aspect of telemedicine. Some of these questions are as follows:

1. Will telemedicine minimize health service cost?
2. Is investment in telemedicine more profitable than investing in other health care systems?
3. Which element of telemedicine is more profitable (if it is indeed so)— the service suppliers, the consumer, or the medical insurance institutions?
4. Is the level of improvement in medical service gained from telemedicine higher than the level of financial investment required?
5. Is it now possible to discuss the profitability of investing in telemedicine, or is telemedicine technology still too expensive and unreliable?

There are still no firm answers to these and other questions, although during the past few years a number of projects have been carried out showing positive economic results in this area.

Calculation of telemedicine service costs must take into consideration expenditure on hardware, software, ongoing expenses of network service, standard upkeep costs, and manpower. Less tangible but no less important, costs such as time required to study the new system, and inconvenience to service suppliers during adaptation to new work locations must be considered as well. In the past, the high cost of software was the major obstacle to setting up telemedicine projects. Today this is not valid, since equipment that in the past required investing $100,000 can be acquired today for less than $15,000.

Until recently few economic evaluations of telemedicine have been performed, as medical insurance institutes only rarely recognize patient expenditure for this kind of medical service.

Economic evaluations that have been performed demonstrated

the following:
- Telemedicine service to rural areas saves $1,000 per patient.
- More profit for service suppliers and less cost to consumer/patients.
- Return of initial investment two to three years into the project.

As mentioned above, the lack of recognition by the medical insurance institutions is a serious obstacle to telemedicine application (Williams & Moore, 1995).

One of the central elements of health service expense is the cost of manpower. This element becomes more costly if the division of responsibility between nurses, doctors and paramedics, is not effective. Doctors, who are a much more expensive manpower source, are doing many tasks that could be accomplished by nurses.

Cunningham, et al (1978) investigated the possibility of using nurses rather than doctors in application of telemedicine. Findings with regard to pediatric medicine showed that 40% of the time diagnosis via closed circuit television allowed nurses to carry out tasks that doctors had done previously.

Two central components affect the success of telemedicine assimilation:
1. Cost
2. Quality of Service

We will focus on the long-term financial aspects of telemedicine.

MACRO-ECONOMIC ANALYSIS:
The medical market is a consumer market, and it is divided into three parts:
1. Medical Insurance Institutes —private and public "Sick Funds"
2. Government and Private Medical Service Suppliers—hospitals, clinics, medical centers and laboratories.
3. Medical Service Consumers—patients insured and private patients.

The medicine 'market' is not a 'free market' but rather a 'price takers' market. Service suppliers are certainly not going to pressure the private/public Sick Funds to lower prices for patients, as that would also affect their profits. Thus the final price demanded from the

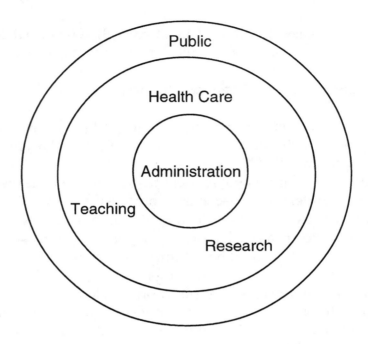

patient is high.

Bodies Profiting from Resulting Saving
1. Medical service suppliers (physicians and nurses).
2. Clinics, medical centers and hospitals.
3. The patient.
4. Medical insurance suppliers (who pay for medical expenses of the medical centers and clinics).
5. Society as a whole

Medical Insurance Suppliers—In the U.S.A. the government foots the bill for telemedicine costs. Therefore, the guiding question regarding costs is whether telemedicine reduces government spending on public health. The government was worried by the possibility that telemedicine would actually raise the cost of government spending on medical services because more patients would demand a specialist opinion. To evaluate this issue the government supplied funding for four research studies in California, Virginia, Ohio, and Iowa to determine whether telemedicine was justified economically, and to decide how to transfer funds to medical service suppliers for telemedicine consultations.

The various studies show that organizations not in need of the support of the medical insurance institutions, such as the U.S. Army, the government health institutes, medical pension plans, and medical institutes in the private sector, adopted telemedicine without apprehension.

Expenditure Savings

There is potential for saving on travel costs, time savings for the patient, saving in medical manpower, saving by not performing unnecessary tests, and saving in cost as a result of treating illness at an early and usually less expensive stage.

There is a general consensus regarding cost saving for conventional medical expenditures (logistics, treatment and diagnosis).

Creating Profit

Clinics can create profit by "receiving" more patients via telemedicine and offering medical supervision of treatment via telemedicine. Additional profit can be derived from the sale of bandwidth to other clinics.

Non-tangible profit that is difficult to calculate: improved trust in village medical services and villagers confidence in those services, resulting in more profit and an assurance of their continuing profitable performance.

Three main telemedicine applications are:
- Medical Consultation
- Medical Instruction
- Management Systems

Medical Consultation

Medical consultation via telemedicine permits the physician to "receive" more patients during a given time, thus creating more profit.

In areas of medicine such as telepathology and teleradiology, utilizing telemedicine in the transfer of visual digital information permits clinicians to support a larger number of patients, both in and outside the clinic.

The clinics can sell and rent out bandwidth to smaller, rural clinics that prefer visual data transfer by communication channels than sending patients to specialists in medical centers. This is less expensive for the patients, and requires less treatment time by the clinic. Thus telemedicine gives the patients more assurance, makes them more loyal, and guarantees the continued existence of rural medical clinics.

Telemedicine can reduce pressure on physicians by replacing them with nurses supported by communication channels and teleconferencing connected to medical centers and physicians. Results of research carried out in New York shows that nurses can function without medical supervision 40% of the time, and expense for installing the required network is two-thirds of the cost of hiring a physician who supplies supervision 100% of the time.

The earliest research on telemedicine consultation, which was carried out by Mueller in 1997 and Marshall Glazer in 1978, examined the subject of cost reduction resulting from using fewer physicians in a workforce made up of nurses and interns, connected via television communication lines to a medical center. According to Mueller, assigning a physician full time to a medical center for the sole purpose of supervision is a waste of funds, as the physician is not occupied the majority of the time.

In 1996 research was done to ascertain if doctors on emergency room duty could be replaced with nurses supervised by telemedicine.

Also, early research in 1975 by Dohner and by Conrath in 1977, revealed that the desirability of the various technologies in communication is identical, and the one preferred was, of course, the most inexpensive – the telephone.

As opposed to this, up-to-date research has shown that the basic cost per system site is $ 50,000, and that cost is justified by 100 hours of use per year (Global Telemedicine Report, 1997).

The Medical Communication Network in Montana reports that a site that supplies 20 medical consultants each month in dermatology, orthopedics, and psychiatry, saves an estimated $ 200 per patient for consultation, while a single consultation saved $ 3,500 in cost for an air ambulance.

A program at the Georgia Medical College revealed that approximately 81% of patients treated via telemedicine did not require examination and treatment from a second or third medical source. In Georgia the difference between cost per bed at a central health center or a rural one is $800. Savings were also reported due to fewer hospitalization days as a result of early treatment, and higher employee productivity. One additional patient at a health center will result in a $150,000 cash flow per year.

Research carried out in Austin, Texas, revealed a minimum of 14% savings in standard physician services. According to the model, reduction in indirect cost and travel time were the central aspects of savings resulting from teleconferencing (an estimated $ 131.6 million in the entire United States). During a period of two years 2,696 patients received treatment, the lives of six patients were saved, and the time necessary for return of funds invested in equipment was three and a half years. An Austin, Texas, specialists clinic reported a profit of $9,000 in the first quarter, a relative cost-profit margin of 2 - 25, and an investment return time of 2.2 years.

In 1992, the University of Texas Tech HealthNet submitted financial records for review by an independent accounting firm of the cost of a telemedicine project. The accounting firm compared the cost of using conventional health services and telemedicine services. Cost savings using Telemedicine was $1,500 per patient. Most savings stemmed from a reduction in the cost of medical treatment as a result of better utilization of less expensive, local medical services, and fewer ambulance services.

Medical Instruction

The expense of medical instruction includes the cost of acquiring teleconferencing equipment and accompanying instruments such as cameras and microphones, installation cost, communication cost, the cost of hiring manpower, manpower instruction cost, equipment maintenance and other indirect costs.

Savings

Cost savings result from less travel time; time spent without gain from the medical aspect. Cost on travel time is saved because the patient can remain at home to receive professional medical instruction. It should be mentioned that in small clinics, the lack of supporting physicians could necessitate the hiring of temporary manpower.

Profit

Professional medical training via telemedicine has resulted in profits from the sale of bandwidth, and has encouraged external bodies to train on site and supply professional training to remote sites.

There are also profits that are not tangible and cannot be quantified such as: profits resulting from professional expertise, enriching the telemedicine databank, improving patient confidence in the quality of medical service, avoiding closure of medical centers, decreasing professional isolation of medical teams at rural medical centers, and maintaining professional manpower.

In any case, researchers feel that instruction via videoconference takes up less time, is better planned and more precise than other means of instruction, and permits more advanced medical instruction.

The Billing Center in Montana supplies instruction to five communities in western Montana, including advanced study programs for physicians, nurse assistants, and other medical suppliers. One hundred and three study programs were carried out in the first year. Saving in cost per participant was $175,000. This factor was calculated on the basis of airfare prices and physician fee, per hour, dissipated on flight time, hotel and food.

The University of Texas Health Center reported that the supply of medical instruction and education via videoconference is a source of profit for the university, supplying programs for 90 sites, 450 hours of instruction to 1,500 medical specialists.

At Texas A&M University a trial was carried out which included 62 physicians and eight classes, showing a savings of $17,000.

Utilizing Telemedicine in Management Systems
Cost saving using telemedicine in management systems is widely documented and is generally applied in organizations controlling a large number of sites. Utilization of telemedicine for management includes: managing conferences by videoconferencing, interviewing candidates, quality control discussions, and manager training while saving travel cost and time. Profit is also generated by videoconferencing for external bodies.

Examples of Telemedicine Utilization in Management
The Baxter Corporation supplies 100,000 products to medical suppliers in 100 countries worldwide. Baxter Corp. holds management conferences via telemedicine, and collaborates with external bodies regarding research via telemedicine. Baxter Corp. reported

savings in travel cost, increased productivity, less time required for decision making, and an increased competitive edge.

HBO & Co. supplies computerized information systems and services to 3,500 hospitals worldwide. The company reported a savings of $ 200,000 in travel time and costs for 3,888 employees, utilization of teleconference interviews, video recording of conferences and transfer to parties interested in the company.

Calculating Telemedicine Expense

Basic Costs
- Equipment purchase (basic, multiplexes, cameras, supplementary instruments and video equipment)
- Communication lines T-1 fixed monthly cost
- Manpower
- Instruction and adaptation
- Installation
- Maintenance

Cost of Medical Consultation
Saving:
1st.   If Physician Travels to Patient
- Cost for specialist and travel time
- Travel expense/flight expense
- Basic consultation time/per hour, hotels, food, loss of work time

2nd.   If Patient Is Brought to Physician
- Ambulance or air-ambulance
- Medical treatment and hospitalization

Cost of Medical Instruction
Savings:
- Travel time saved multiplied by the hourly fee for doctor, specialist, or nurse.
- Employee savings: flight fare, hotels, food and ground travel time

Cost to Management for Telemedicine
Savings:
- Work time for management employees

- Travel time
- Airfare, ground travel time, food and hotels
- Time and money, for candidates who must travel to interview

Financial Summary and Conclusions

As opposed to other areas where, in the future, information sources will completely replace a large portion of the organizational resources, the area of medicine can only integrate information technology as a support system and basically as a solution to logistic problems. Information technologies in medicine will mainly improve the process of supplying medical service. Economic aspects are decisive in every decision regarding acquisition of information technology.

Today medical insurance companies in the U.S.A have only begun to recognize telemedicine as a part of the "medicine service basket." Full recognition by these insurance institutions will make telemedicine available to all patients who need it and not only a few wealthy patients.

TELEMEDICINE INFLUENCE ON SOCIETY AND HEALTH SYSTEMS

- Considerable improvement of the administrative aspect of health systems.
- Medical professionals will have improved access to rapid, high quality and easily assimilated information and data relevant to diagnosis and treatment.
- Physicians will have easy access to second opinion consultation and support in decision making. Instant communication with specialists at large medical centers.
- Bringing communication services into the patient's home will create communication pathways to receive on-the-spot emergency medical treatment. The possibility of immediate communication at the onset of the medical problem will reduce time for diagnosis and treatment (a central factor in emergency medicine). In addition to diagnosis and treatment, the subject of medical instruction and education will also be more accessible to the individual.

- The physical location of medical professionals will cease to be an obstacle in receiving medical instruction and education.
- Improved medical services in areas where the quality of medicine is poor can be achieved by a more homogenous allocation of medical services on the clinical communication network.
- Considerable loosening of the bureaucracy knot currently weighing down the medical system. Approaching and solving management problems via the home computer.
- Medical information systems, with improved methods for gathering, storing and receiving data, will facilitate effective transfer of knowledge from research level to assimilation and application level. A large amount of factual information will be available and can be utilized in research.
- Improve the decision-making process governing managerial and policy decisions, situation assessment and planning, by means of information-gathering tools, deciphering and disseminating the information.
- Finally, we expect heightened competition between medical service suppliers, which will result from the lack of need for physical proximity between physician and patient.

In general, it can be assumed that the above-mentioned improvements are a suitable reason to deal with and overcome the major obstacles to developing and applying telemedicine.

Telemedicine acceptance in the daily life of the individual and into organizational proceedings will mandate a profound change in clinical and organizational concepts. There will be a real revolution in the organic structure of accepted health systems.

The central and most important development is the partial cancellation of the geographical factor in supplying health services. Bringing the patient to the doctor and the doctor to the patient via telemedicine, shortening response time and quality top level communication between the involved bodies, will all play an important part in a widespread solution to the worldwide health supply system crisis.

MEDICAL RECORDS ON THE INFORMATION NETWORK – CENTRAL ISSUES

A basic and central element of telemedicine is the computer-based patient record. This subject has been widely discussed in the medical world and is a central topic in the reform plans of American health systems. The computerized and network-assimilated medical record should be comparatively accessible, reliable and cheap. It is difficult today to find any ongoing dialogue which questions the benefit of switching from conventional filing to computerized filing. The use of computerized filing is usually an accepted given and dialogue will be focused on questions relating to application and the consequences.

For the present, however, at least in Israel, there is no centralized filing system for medical files. Each patient has medical files and parts of medical files scattered at different locations such as clinics, hospitals, and private clinics; a large amount of paper work with very little computerized medical information (such as laboratory results).

This part of the chapter looks at a short survey we've done of five social and organizational issues related to computerized, network-assimilated medical records.

1. Who's "property" is the medical file?
2. Who is in possession of the medical file?
3. How can the patient's "right to privacy" be maintained while still making important medical data available?
4. Should medical service suppliers have access to medical files?
5. Should indepth access to medical files be allowed and what system should be utilized to do so?

In closing, we shall endeavor to put forth a possible resolution of the problem under discussion, as expressed in the British Medical Associations' Medical Information Security Principles (Anderson, 1996).

Whose "Property" Is the Medical File?

Ownership of medical file information is still not fully regulated in law, nor do acceptable unwritten laws governing this issue exist. Forming new information properties, such as computer-based medical files for the population, requires a dialogue regarding ownership. For the purpose of the dialogue, we shall offer five main possibilities:

1. Each citizen owns his or her medical file.
2. The body that compiles the medical file owns it (the dental clinic where the patients x-rays were carried out owns the medical file containing those x-rays).

3. Medical service supplier.
4. A central medical service supplier (Kupat Holim, for example) will own the entire medical file.
5. The medical file would be the property of The Medical Insurance Institute.

The logical assumption should be that the medical file is the property of the individual patient; however, in a new information age, this question gains more meaning than ever before. When medical data is held in paper files, medical information suppliers cannot effectively utilize it.

If medical data is electrically transferable and accessible in large quantities, it will then be of great interest to medical information suppliers, beginning with aggregated information management and operation needs, including sale of data for aggregation and perhaps even for individual purposes (data mining for pharmaceutical companies). The medical insurer has an important vested interest in medical information: maintaining the reliability and perfection of information that may be imperative in preventing expenditure, and gathering a complete medical picture that can effect the pricing of medical insurance. Finally, it is still in the individual's best interest (perhaps now more than in the past) to have ownership of his medical file. Ownership will render him less dependent on medical service suppliers or medical insurance institutes of one kind or another, and will permit him or her to benefit from heightened competition between these organizations.

Any decision regarding these questions on which the various possibilities for medical file ownership shall be adopted (perhaps a combination of one or more possibilities) will, undoubtedly, be influenced by ethnic factors, political factors, and financial arguments put forth by each of the interested invested parties. One possibility, stemming from the recommendations of the British Medical Association, is that each individual shall own his medical file.

In Whose "Physical" Trust Should the Medical File Remain?

When the dilemma regarding ownership of the computer-based medical file has been resolved, it will then remain to be decided in whose " physical" possession the file will remain. In the era of paper filing the file would have remained at the medical service supplier, or the insurer's premises. In the era of the *information highway*, the individual may have possession of his medical file (for example at his own Web site), and he could then permit access to the suppliers and insurers. It may be preferable, however, for medical files to be stored in central locations thus maintaining quality, accessibility and security. Central sites could be the medical service suppliers, the medical insurer, or at companies specializing in storing information and not connected to a particular medical insurance institute or the specific patient. Because the subject under discussion is an information package, and not a physical object, several copies may exist (*mirror sites*) at different locations held by different bodies, or the information may be divided up by subject and held at several different locations.

The solution which seems to be indicated by the British Medical Association, for example, is that the medical service suppliers hold the file of medical information. The Association opposes the suggestion that the medical insurance institutes, the medical service suppliers, or the National Health Service have possession of the file, because their facilities do not sufficiently protect the patient's *"right to privacy."*

Patients "Right to Privacy" Versus Accessing Essential Medical Data

Along with the decision regarding ownership of medical files, decisions must be made regarding access to files and secrecy of the files contents.

Medical files contain a variety of medical data and types of medical information that demand a different level of consideration with regard to information security. The variety of information contained in the medical file ranges from information that the patient would, most likely, not mind being divulged (identifying marks, childhood diseases, inoculations, and blood type), to information that the patient would certainly not want divulged (doctors' notes from office visits, different treatments), and even contains information that could be considerably harmful to the individual (information regarding past psychological disturbances and evaluation of potential for mental illness).

The *"right to privacy"* is a central patient issue. This is demonstrated by Skolnick, who maintains that the quality and effectiveness of the relationship between the individual and the medical system depends on the individual being assured that his "Right to Privacy" is guaranteed. A situation wherein security of medical files is not guaranteed, may result in the patient withholding important medical data (physicians may resort to this as well), and an even more extreme result, the creation of a medical service market that does not computerize data. Because a promise of *privacy* on the network is, in his opinion, not practical, Skolnick proposes that each individual have possession of his medical file (Skolnick, 1994).

Despite the need for individual privacy, situations do exist where at least a part of the information deserves to be made public. That is to say, a trade-off exists between the privacy level and the discovery level. In cases of accidents, immediate revelation of medical information to the treating medical team (teams' identity is unknown beforehand) can mean the difference between life and death. Beyond that, in case of an accident, the one in possession of the medical information may be the victim, and if he or she is, for example unconscious, he or she may not be able to answer questions or give access codes to the information to receive lifesaving treatment. Of particular interest to us is the fact that, even if we limit our consideration only to the individual, we conclude that the issue of *"right to privacy"* is not of supreme importance.

The subject of the individual's *"right to privacy"* is discussed in detail in the recommendation of the British Medical Association. Mechanisms such as access lists and audit trails are suggested, as well as coding and electronic signatures, to insure security of network information, and removing restrictions during emergencies.

Should Non-Medical Service Suppliers Have Indepth Access to Medical Files?

Medical information is of interest to different bodies aside from service suppliers: government bodies such as the Police Department and Social Services; private financial bodies such as potential employers, insurance institutes, credit banks; or commercial bodies such as pharmaceutical companies.

For example, Woodward is apprehensive of allowing access to bodies such as potential employers, insurers and educational institutes who may use the information in a prejudicial manner. As an illustration Woodward sites the Computer-Based Patient Record Institute, supported by organizations dealing in medical services, insurance, and information systems. These programs also allow "access to information for reasons other than those directly related to medical treatment." Woodward is also concerned by the fact that the organizations and government agencies involved in medical service plan to allow themselves access to information and perceive this as a threat to "medical supervision" of the individual (Woodward, 1995).

It is an accepted idea that this approach will bar private financial bodies from medical files, but how it will effect access by government agencies is less clear.

The British Medical Association demands that no one other than the patient or his treating physician be granted access and that other organizations receive handwritten information only. It defines the National Health Service information network as unethical, because it allows access by government and state agencies.

When and How to Permit Constrained Access to Medical Files

Some doubt the supreme value of the *"right to medical privacy"* and cite the concept of *public information*. Arguments are usually made from a social point of view. Gathering of authentic information from numerous medical files can be used in medical research that will improve individual welfare and the welfare of society as a whole. Discovery can result from an anonymous request by the medical file's owner, thus minimizing any harm as far as privacy is concerned. On the other hand, it will be possible to identify patients without the need for direct access to their name, i.e., by cross-referencing information.

For example, Gostin maintains that modern society should not elevate individual privacy above the interests of society. He believes that constrained gathering of information is an essential part of reforming health systems (Gostin, 1995). A different approach, financial rather than ethical, offers a possible way to retrieve constrained information. Laudon suggests creating information markets where individuals could *"sell"* medical information from their files to pharmaceutical companies, for example Laudon (1996).

The recommendations of the British Medical Association call for the patient to be alerted if a person whose name has been suggested as an addition to the list of people with access to his file, already has access to a large number of medical files.

British Medical Association Recommendations

The question raised in the previous paragraphs are referred to and receive at least a partial answer in the Security of Medical Information Principles of the British Medical Association (Anderson, 1996). We present these principles here as one example of a possible way to deal with the computer-based medical file.

1. Access Control – An access list of those persons or organizations authorized access to the file, or authorized to add information to the file, will be attached to each file.

2. Record Opening – Only persons or organizations on the access list will have access.

3. Control – One of the medical staff whose name appears on the access list will be responsible, and only he or she will be allowed to change the access list or add professional medical comments to the file.

4. Consent and Notification – The medical staff member chosen to be responsible, must inform the patient of the names appearing on the access list, and any change that is made. Except in emergencies, the patient must be consulted before any change is made.

5. Persistence – No data can be erased in any case.

6. Attribution – The file will contain a record of who has accessed the file, including name, date and time.

7. Information Flow – Data from one file may be entered into a second file, only if a copy of the access list from the second file is added to the access list of the first file.

8. Aggregation Control – Measures will be taken to prevent aggregation of private medical data. In particular the patient should be alerted if a person, whose name has been suggested as an addition to the access list, is already on the access list of a large number of medical files.

9. Trusted Computing Base – A computer system that handles private medical information must have a subsystem capable of applying the aforementioned principles.

We have reviewed five issues related to computer-based medical files and have given one example of a possible solution to the questions these issues raise. We do not surmise to say that these are a total of all of the social and organizational issues, and there are, obviously, other answers to the questions these issues raise. It seems to us, however, that our dialogue demonstrates the effect a change in the information systems will have on the individual, on the organizational level, and on society as a whole.

The issue of "ownership" of the medical file will affect the balance of power between the individual, the medical service supplier, the health insurance institutes, and the other players on the medical field. The issues of "physical possession" of the medical file will profoundly affect the way medical service suppliers are organized, their measure of autonomy, and the connection between physicians and the large medical centers.

In addition, companies dealing in storage of medical information have begun to appear in the United States. The "privacy" issue is affected by and in turn affects the two previous issues of "ownership" and "physical possession" of medical files, and in addition have meaning regarding problem-solving technologies, in competition between storing medical files on a network or storing them on smart cards. Finally, the last two issues of access by external bodies to medical files and gathering restricted information from the file, will have an effect on society from an economic point of view, as well as from the point of view of medical research.

TELEMEDICINE TECHNOLOGY

The term telemedicine refers to medical information transferred through modern communication. These two ancient words *medicine* and *communication* where first linked at the beginning of the 20th century, when ships used radio communication to receive medical assistance, however, only in the early 1960s did that link become truly significant. When we discuss communication from the technological aspect, we refer to the means permitting widespread transfer of information.

There is a clear and obvious correlation between technological development, in communication and other technological areas, such as image compression and adaptation, storage, and robotics, and advances in medical service in communication.

Initially, microwaves were used to transfer information. Later on satellites were used to transmit information. This resulted mainly from NASA entering the medical communication arena. The majority of the information transferred was static: x-rays, laboratory results, etc. After the advent of satellite communication, visual information such as video images and, later on, images and results were transferred directly from the medical instrument.

At the same time, improved technologies for information transfer were developed. Image compression and adaptation are just a couple examples.

Medicine in Communication via Mobile Satellite

With the goal of supplying paramedic services via automated vehicles, medical technology was introduced to transmit data via satellite communications.

Utilizing this technology, diagnosis and emergency treatment by a specialist may be performed on the spot, with no time wasted.

Typical problems involved in this technique are:
* Channel overload
* System size
* Credibility of transfer of vital signs
* Real-time action
* Electromagnetic communication

Perimeters have been set for these problems, and their effectiveness has been analyzed. A defined data structure and an experimental system have been developed.

The system can transmit color images, voice signals, three channel EEG and blood pressure simultaneously from a mobile station to a ground station. The system can also transmit voice signals and signals to prevent errors from the ground station to the mobile station via full duplex, and finally, experimental broadcasts of medical information by a ship at sea or an airplane on an international flight course.

C/N (o) value limit measured to ensure valid receipt of information was much lower that the lowest C/N (o) value limit for communication. As a result technical application of this technique was validated (Muraakami,1994).

Transfer of Laboratory Images

In April 1986, Murphy and Bird investigated 1,000 cases of medicine in communication between the Massachusetts General Hospital (MGH) and the Logan International Airport, who utilized non-color cameras, connected to a microscope, in transmitting images of blood and urine tests via microwave transmission.

In August 1986, in El Paso, Texas, a video of a microscope robot was first presented when Dr. Ronald S. Washington presented images of a chest biopsy, which were transmitted via satellite connection from Washington. Two basic types of pathology in communication are involved in low-cost transfer of static images, using the "Save" and "Send" (SAF) and the Interactive and Dynamic Video (IATV).

In certain systems the robot controls the system. At a system in Wake Forrest, North Carolina (an example of a experimental system), the finding of the system during the course of this experiment, and those reached by standard pathology were compatible 95% of the time (Seykora, 1995).

Quality Analyzing Compressed Medical Images

Compression of digital images can result in more efficient transmission, storage and adaptation of images. As radiology departments transfer to greater digital technology, the amount of images will result in a demand for more utilization of systems for image compression (picture archiving and communication systems (PACS) and *teleradiology* systems).

Significant image compression can only be achieved by the use of unstable algorithms that do not permit precise reconstruction of the original image. There is disagreement regarding this loss of information because there is a potential of image loss and related problems of image sharpness. This technology must, however, be given consideration, because the alternative is delay, damage, and loss of communication and return of information.

How do we decide if an image is of high enough quality to be used for diagnosis, archive reconstruction from archive, or study purposes?

The tests to determine quality of medical images is threefold:
• Signal - noise ratio
• Subject grading
• Precision of diagnosis (Cosman, Gray and Olshen , 1994).

Technological Considerations In Planning Decentralized Teleradiology

A wide spectrum teleradiology project is now underway to connect an image center in Florida to the UCLA Radiology Department. The goal is to supply patients in Florida with routine medical treatment utilizing consultation from the academic radiology department.

The project is expected to expand and include local and international locations.

Technologies involved in planning the achievement of a teleradiology infrastructure will handle network planning, image compression, decentralized archives and special viewing stations.

Special emphasis will be placed on planning an archive that will make intelligent use of information, such as activating events from a Radiology Information System (RIS).

Terms such as long distance consultation and long distance procedure guidance and control are aimed at supplying the same high-level quality medical services to rural areas as to densely populated areas. (Ho, Taira, Steckel and Kangarloo , 1995).

Applying Advanced Telemedicine

Incite, a company based in Dallas, Texas, has uncovered a new *telemedicine* application called *MedCite*. The application is based on a conversational media platform, and its aim is to give the medical community multimedia decentralized capabilities based on the network. As of December 1, 1996, MedCite bases its integral capabilities on Conversational Media that includes special switchboards, an advanced multimedia server, and customer software and hardware.

MedCite will be more intuitive in medical surroundings. Incite includes a table that is capable of capturing images that will give the systems the capability to transmit S-Video from medical instruments to allow diagnosis and pick up, transmit, and share high quality images from invasive cameras, microscopic video, CT Scan, and other medical equipment. The system has the capabilities for storage and transmission that allow the physicians to record vocal multimedia pulses, video, images and statistics, and transfer them to colleagues for consultation, in a service similar to electronic mail.

According to David Tucker, CEO of Incite, "MedCite brings down the geographical boundaries of medical treatment service, makes unusual medical treatment more accessible and feasible to even the most remote areas" (*Business Wire*, October 18, 1996).

This era is a fascinating one from the standpoint of Technologies. The rate of technological development, particularly in the field of computers and information systems, is the most rapid that humanity has witnessed.

We hear of new developments in computer software, hardware,

and communication. We think that medicine in communication, propelled by technological innovations, will advance and broaden existing applications.

Today the concept of *virtual reality* is in its infancy, but we envision a time when it will play a significant role in the field of medicine, and medicine in communication. Virtual reality can be utilized in the instruction of physicians regarding complicated procedures and operations, or to treat rare cases, thus improving the physician's skills. Another possible application is operations performed by a robot, guided by a physician at an entirely different location. Despite the distance dividing the different locations, the physician will "see" the patient and make the gestures required for the procedure, and the robot will "copy" those gestures.

Along with other technological advances, "smart agents" and optimum reduction will make it possible to put electrodes on a patient, transmit data such as hormone levels to the medical center where the patient is being treated, and receive recommendations for treatment.

The wise and accurate use of "smart cards" containing all the patients' medical information, and the advances in the development of image compression techniques, may result in the inclusion of x-rays and other visual data on those cards.

When the project, the goal of which is mapping all human genes, and the forming of a worldwide human gene database, is completed, it will be possible to determine a person's chances of carrying a gene for an inherited disease or to perform a precise evaluation of diseases.

Systems supplying specialist consultations at various levels will be able to provide consultations regarding specific problems in distant areas not accessible to the physician specialist himself.

LOOKING INTO THE FUTURE

In the near future, even if new developments occur in the course of removing obstacles to the advancement of telemedicine, expansion of the already massive entrance to the *information highway* of its various applications is not expected.

To perceive telemedicine as a part of the national or international *information highway* rather than a 'golf course for the privileged', or as an 'academic pathway,' it must have practical recognition by the state and/or medical insurance institutes as an integral part of the total 'medical services basket.'

We cannot ignore other obstacles standing in the way of advance, even if it is easier to assume that problems related to the various information technologies, such as patients 'right to privacy', cost versus effectivity findings, etc., will be solved in the near future.

It is agreed that in the future the field of telemedicine will become central to and an integral part of the *information highway*, assuming that the many problems and obstacles existing are identified and effectively dealt with.

In order not to follow a "prophet of fools" we will not attempt to forecast the time, place, or means for telemedicine implementation. However, we will try to describe the way it will influence the individual, the organization and the social structure as a whole, assuming that telemedicine is transformed into a practical and viable part of every day life.

Telemedicine influence on the individual:
- Substantial improvement in the administrative systems of health systems.
- Improved accessibility of physicians (in terms of speed, quality, and effectiveness) to medical information and data relevant to diagnosis .
- Better physician access to *second opinion* advice, and more support in the decision-making process. Fast, immediate communication with specialist at large medical centers.
- Bringing information services into the individuals home will create opportunities for split-second receipt of primary emergency medical treatment via new communication technologies. Diagnosis and treatment of appearing medical problems will be immediate (a perimeter central to emergency medicine). Besides medical treatment and diagnosis, medical education and instruction will be more accessible to the individual.
- The geographical location of the medical staff will cease to be an obstacle to professional medical education.
- Improved medical service in areas where the quality of medicine is inferior, resulting from a more homogeneous allocation of medical services on the clinical information network.
- Less bureaucracy in medicine. Management problems and solutions on the home computer.

- By improving systems for aggregation, storage and receipt of information, medical information systems will be able to transfer information from the research level to the dissemination level more effectively. Large quantities of accurate information will become available for research.
- Improved management and decision-making processes, planning and estimates by means of information aggregation instruments, their evaluation and dissemination.
- Finally, we envision increased competition in supply of medical services, resulting from the fact that the physical location of the physician and the patient will cease to be of importance.

In general we can assume that the above improvements are a substantial enough reason to require us to deal with and remove the majority of the obstacles standing in the path of the advancement of telemedicine.

Acceptance of telemedicine in the life of the individual and the organization will demand a substantial change in clinical and organizational conceptions, and will result in a revolution in the existing accepted health organization structure, in treatment and diagnosis procedures, and in the health system policy as a whole.

REFERENCES

Anderson, R.(1996). Clinical system security: interim guidelines. *British Medical Journal*, 13 Jan.

Baer, L., et al. (1995). Pilot studies of telemedicine for patients with obsessive-compulsive disorder. *Am J Psychiatry*, Sep.

Bashshur R. (1978). Public acceptance of telemedicine in a rural community. *Biosci. Commun.* 4: 17-38.

Bashshur, R. (1980). Technology serves the people; the story of a cooperative telemedicine project by NASA, the Indian Health Service and the Papago people. Superintendent of Documents, US. Government Printing Office, Washington, DC: 1-110.

Bashshur, R. and Lovett, J. (1977). Assessment of telemedicine: results of the initial experience. *Aviat. Space Environ. Med.* 48(1): 65-70.

Bashshur, R.L., Armstrong PA and Youssef Z I (1975). *Telemedicine; Explorations in the use of telecommunications in health care.* Charles C. Thomas, Springfield, IL: 1-356.

Benschoter, R. A. (1971). CCTV-Pioneering Nebraska Medical Center. *Educational Broadcasting* : 1-3.

Business Wire , October 18, 1996

Campion E. (1995). New hope for home care? (Editorial). *New England Journal of Medicine* 333(18): 1213-1214.

Cosman, P.C., Gray, R.M. and Olshen, R.A. (1994). Evaluating quality of compressed medical images. *Proceedings of the IEEE*: 919-932

Cunningham, N., Marshall, C., & Glazer, E. (1978, December 15). Telemedicine in   pediatric primary care. *JAMA*, 240(25), 2749-2751.

Eide, T.J., et al. (1994). Current status of telepathology. *APMIS*, December.

Engstrom, P. (1996). Telemedicine targets a rapid-growth market: home sweethome care. *Medicine on the Net* 2(5): 1-4.

Foote, D.R. (1977) Satellite communication for rural health care in Alaska. *J. Commun.* 27(4): 173-182.

Furtado, R. (1982, March). Telemedicine: The next-best thing to being there. *Dimensions*, 10-12.

Goldberg, M.A., et al. (1994). Making global telemedicine practical and affordable: demonstrations from the Middle East. (*AJR Am J Roentgenol*, December.

Gostin L. O., Health information privacy, *Cornell Law Review*, 1995.

Hartman, J. T., & Moore, M. (1992). Using telecommunications to improve rural healthcare: The Texas Tech MEDNET Demonstration Project. Prepared for the Office of Rural Health Policy, U.S. Department of Health and Human Services. Lubbock: Texas Tech University.

House, M. (1991). Canadian experience: using telemedicine for the support of medical care at remote sites. NASA, Washington, International Telemedicine/Disaster Medicine Conference.

Kavanagh, S.J., et al.(1995). Telemedicine—clinical applications in mental health. *Aust Fam Physician*, July.

Korsoff, L., et al. (1995). Experiences with a teleradiology system in pulmonary diseases.*Acta Radiol*, January.

Laudon, K. C. (1996). Markets and privacy, *Communications of the ACM*, Sept.

Moore, M. (1993a). Elements of success in telemedicine projects. Report of a research grant from AT&T; Graduate School of Library and Information Science, the University of Texas at Austin.

Muller, C., Marshall, C.L., Krasner, M., Cunningham, N., Wallerstein, E., & Thomstad, B. (1977). Cost factors in urban telemedicine. *Medical Care*,15(3), 251-259.

Muraakami, H., et al.(1994). Telemedicine using mobile satellite communication. *IEEE Transaction on biomedicine Engineering*, 41(5), 488 - 497

Murphy, R.L.J. and Bird, K.T. (1974). Telediagnosis: a new community health resource; observations on the feasibility of telediagnosis based on 1000 patient transactions. *Am. J. Public Health* 64(2): 113-119.

Peters, T. (1988). *Thriving on chaos*. New York: Harper & Row.

Seykora, P. .J (1995). Background to telepathology. *Telemedicine Today* 3(4): 18-20,29.

Siwicki, B. (1996). The home care market offers telemedicine opportunities. *Health Data Management* 4(5): 52-56

Skolnick, A. A. (1994). Protecting privacy of computerized patient information may lie in the cards, *Journal of the American Medical Association*, July 20.

Williams, F. & Moore, M. (1995). Telemedicine: its place on the information highway.

Woodward, B. (1995). The computer-based patient record and confidentiality, *The New England Journal of Medicine*, Nov. 23.

Wright R., et al. (1995). Teleradiology. *BM*, May 27.

Chapter X

Client-Server Computing: Lessons Learned and an Application in the Healthcare Industry

Mahesh S. Raisinghani
University of Dallas, USA

Ann Shou-an Char
Parkland (TX) Health & Hospital System, USA

INTRODUCTION

Client-server architecture is a local area network (LAN) based computing environment in which a central database sever or engine performs all database commands sent to it from client workstations, and application programs on each client concentrate on user interface functions. Client-server computing is a phrase used to describe a model for computer networking. In this shared processing model, a server has an intelligent database engine functioning as a service on the network. This model offers an efficient way to provide data/ information and services to many users as needed. A network connection is only made when a user needs to access the information or obtain the needed service. This lack of a continuous network connection provides network efficiency. Any change made in the server is transparent to clients.

A client is a requester for networked data/information and service. A client is usually a personal computer (PC) or a workstation that can query a database and/or other information from a server. Typical client functions are to display the user interface, perform basic input editing, format queries to be forwarded to the server processor, communicate with the server, and format server responses for presentation.

A server is a computer that stores information for manipulation by networked clients. Examples of servers are a mainframe, a high powered workstation/PC, or a minicomputer. A server is passive and it does not initiate conversations with clients although it can act as a client of other servers. A server waits for and accepts clients, presents a defined abstract interface to clients, and maintains the location independence and transparency of client interface.

A client/server system allows one or more clients to request data from one or more servers and put the data to a convenient place for clients. An underlying operating system and inter-process communication system are required to form a composite system for distributing computation, analysis, and presentation.

CHARACTERISTICS OF CLIENT-SERVER COMPUTING

The major characteristics of a client-server include the logical separation of the client processes from the server processes, as well as the ability to change a client without affecting the server or other clients. Client-server computing is distinct from ordinary distributed processing. There is a heavy reliance on bringing user-friendly applications to the user's front-end system. The client-based station generally represents the type of graphical interface that is most comfortable to users. This gives the user a great deal of control over the timing and computer uses and gives department-level managers the ability to be responsive to their local needs.

When the applications are dispersed, there is an emphasis on centralizing corporate databases and many network management and utility functions. This enables management to maintain overall control of the total capital investment in computing and information systems and enables management to provide interoperability so that systems are tied together. At the same time, it relieves individual departments and divisions of much of the overhead of maintaining sophisticated computer-based facilities, but it enables them to choose just about any type of machine and interface they need to access data and information. There is a commitment, both by user organizations and vendors, to open and modular systems, which means that the user has greater choice in selecting products and in mixing equipment from a number of vendors. Networking is fundamental to the operation. Thus, network management and network security have a high priority when planning the design and implementation of healthcare information systems using client-server architecture.

CLIENT-SERVER COMPONENTS

There are three types of client-server architectures, and what makes the client-server system work is the software application process on the client (Vaskevitch, 1997).

Software Architecture

The software architecture comprises three layers of software application. These are the presentation layer, the business logic layer, and the data management layer. Each of these three layers is discussed below.

The presentation layer takes the incoming data from external stimuli and edits it. The language paradigm for this layer is mostly object-oriented nowadays. This layer is almost always located on a client machine, but it is not a strict rule. Some PC's may be used as mainframe screens that it does not keep the origin of the presentation logic. The presentation layer also will present the response from the server to the outside world.

The business logic layer is the heart of the client-server system. The code that executes the business policy, rules, and regulations is in this layer and it can be located on the client, the server, or in between the client and server. The language paradigm for the business logic layer depends on the development tool chosen. It can be a mixed language layer, but the trend is towards object-oriented constructs.

The data management layer is charged with access and corporation of data. When this layer receives the data request, it will read and write the data and send the data to where it was requested. The language paradigm for this layer is normally a relational database. As the need of video, multimedia, sound, and hypertext objects, unstructured data is also collected here.

The overview of the software structure flow can be described as a circular system as indicated in Figure 1. When the presentation layer (a PC) receives an input (data request), it informs the business logic layer to analyze the request to match against the code and search in the data management layer. When the data request is matched in the data management layer, the data is then sent back to the presentation layer through the business logic layer.

Fat Client vs. Thin Client

With a **fat client (thin server)** the client has ability to control the data. The execution is mostly performed on the client machine. The server is responsible for sending data to the client and back to server.

With a **thin client (fat server)** the client is restricted to the presentation layer and the majority of business logic is performed on the server. The first generation of development tools Graphic User Interface (GUI) like Visual Basic and PowerBuilder encouraged two-

Figure 1

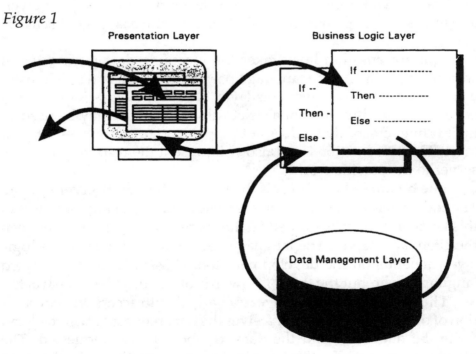

Software layers

Source: Ruble, D. (1997), Practical Analysis and Design for Client/Server & GUI Systems, New Jersey: Prentice Hall, Inc.

tier hardware architecture. The user-friendly development tools enabled the user's presentation performance. The second GUI development tools generation separated presentation from business logic. The characteristics of the second GUI generations are reusable, portable, and maintainable. They promoted the reusability because they are very mechanical in nature. They are portable because they separate presentation and business logic. They are maintainable because business logic is separated and kept in one place so that the change is transparent to both the client and the server.

Hardware Architecture

The software structures do not function alone. The software structures and hardware structures are interdependent on each other. They need each other to make the client-server system function. The hardware architecture comprises a two-tier, three-tier, or an n-tier

Figure 2

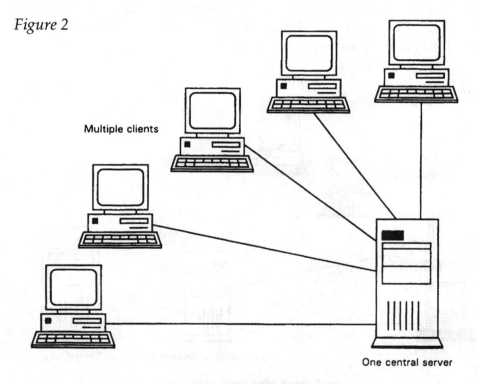

Multiple clients

One central server

A two tier client/server architecture

Source: Ruble, D. (1997), Practical Analysis and Design for Client/Server & GUI Systems, New Jersey: Prentice Hall, Inc.

client-server architecture. The choice among these alternative architectures should be based on the scope and complexity of a project, the time available for completion, and the expected enhancement or obsolescence of the system.

The two-tiered architecture consists of a client and a server where the logic areas are combined on the client as shown in Figure 2. When the client requests data from the server in the two-tiered architecture environment, the software layers concept starts running among the hardware architecture. The presentation and business logic layers take place on the client and the data management layer is as the server. The language paradigm used is typically SQL.

In most cases, a two-tier system can be developed in a small fraction of the time it would take to code a comparable but less-flexible legacy system. It also interacts well with prototyping and Rapid Application Development (RAD) techniques, which can be used to ensure that the requirements of the users are accurately and completely met. Two-tiered architecture works well in environments that have fairly static business rules.

Figure 3

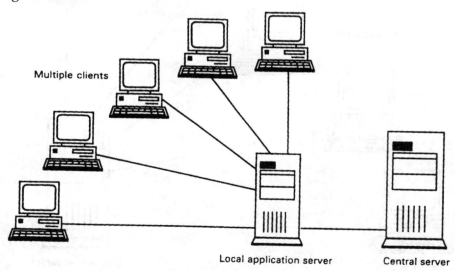

A three tier client/server architecture

Source: Ruble, D. (1997), Practical Analysis and Design for Client/Server & GUI Systems, New Jersey: Prentice Hall, Inc.

When there is a change in business rules, it would require a change to the client logic in each application. System security in the two-tier environment can be complicated because a user may require a separate password for each SQL server accessed. The proliferation of end-user query tools can also compromise database server security. Client tools and the SQL middleware used in two-tier environments are also highly proprietary, and the PC tools market is extremely volatile. The volatility of the client-server tool market raises questions about the long-term viability of any proprietary tool to which an organization may commit, therefore complicating the implementation of two-tier systems.

The three-tier hardware architecture contains clients (presentation layer), local application server (functionality layer), and central server (data management layer). Unlike the two-tier hardware archi-

Figure 4

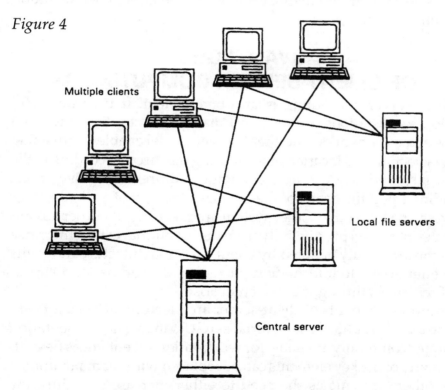

An n-tier client/server architecture

Source: Ruble, D. (1997), Practical Analysis and Design for Client/Server & GUI Systems, New Jersey: Prentice Hall, Inc.

tecture, the software architecture applied to it is logically separated. In the three-tiered architecture there are three logical and distinct application, i.e., the data management, presentation and analysis which are combined to create a single information system.

It is important to note that in the three-tier hardware architecture illustrated in Figure 3, the roles of a client and a central server are the same as in the two-tier hardware architecture, but the role of a local application server is not a fixed role. It can be a client to the central server and a server to the clients depending on the direction of communication.

The n-tier client-server architecture is the compound model of the three-tier hardware architecture. It lets the PCs connect directly to the database server and bypass the local server as illustrated in Figure 4. N-tier architecture allows the client and the server to function in a seamless and integrated manner that results in easier customization and maintenance.

ADVANTAGES
OF CLIENT-SERVER COMPUTING

Client-server computing is an open system. It uses powerful graphical workstations, servers, and mainframes to distribute data process across networks. The client-server model enables rightsizing and the selection and location of computing resources according to the individual's and workgroup's changing requirements. Over time, depending upon the needs of the business, the cost of a client-server system can be lower then other system architectures. Another advantage is the increased productivity from the individual to the enterprise due to the autonomy enabled by client-server architecture. It results from better access to information for requesters and better distribution of resources throughout the enterprise.

Additional benefits of client-server architecture include: it facilitates the use of graphical user interfaces (GUI) and visual presentation techniques commonly available for workstations; it enhances flexibility since any of the key elements can be replaced without major impact on the other elements as the need to either increase or reduce the processing for that element dictates; it allows using less expensive processors on each platform to insure cost effectiveness; it facilitates new technology to be incorporated into the system; it facilitates domain, entity, and referential integrity to be maintained on a single database server; it allows most processing to be performed close to the source of processed data, thereby improving response times and reducing network traffic; it allows for and encourages the acceptance of open systems; and it permits data security (only in the application lever) to be centralized on the server (Renauld, 1993).

DISADVANTAGES OF CLIENT-SERVER COMPUTING

There is no right or perfect solution for all businesses on management decision even though client-server computing provides innovative services for a number of businesses. Careful strategic planning is required up front because of the flexibility of the client-server systems and the complexity of networking. Some other disadvantages are:

- The hardware, software, and communications technology is neither mature nor entirely stable, nor easy to assemble.
- Since client-server is not well understood it is frequently sold inappropriately or oversold to management and unsatisfied expectations result.
- Support costs can run three times the price of system hardware and software.
- Redesign and reprogramming are not trivial exercises.
- Backup and recovery in a client-server environment can be expensive.
- The more distributed the network, the greater its vulnerability.
- Client-server is an evolving technology and as such there is no standardization.

Client-server computing allows an organization to rapidly create applications that reflect changing business needs. However, underneath the surface are costs that can make client-sever systems more expensive to operate than centralized host-based systems. Thus, complete life cycle costs and total cost of ownership must be considered.

SOME MYTHS
OF CLIENT-SERVER DEVELOPMENT

There are a number of myths associated with client-server development. Ruble (1997) and Vaskevitch (1997) discuss some of them as follows:

1. *"Client-server technology will make users more productive."*
   Client-server technology can enable users to be more productive because it is usually used to provide information to those who need it. It does not guarantee a greater productivity if one uses client-server systems for business purposes.

2.1 *"Client-server is less expensive."*
   Some people may just look at the hardware cost and forget about the invisible costs like manpower-related costs for reengineering the business and associated training, and loss of long-term employees because they cannot adopt the new system.

2.2 *"We can use the new system to enable improvements in the business process."*
   This statement is persuasive only if the employees are satisfied and can be more productive. Effective software, trained users and supporters, and improved procedures support the business process improvement.

2.3 *"Hardware costs will go down."*
   It is easier to request data by using new software so that more people request more information. This increases the need for processing power which increases costs for the additional hardware needed to respond to the increased demand.

3. *"PC stands for personal computer."*
   Some employees abuse their freedom of access to the Internet or other personal uses. Sometimes these actions damage the PC (the company's property). That is why PC does not stand for personal computer. Therefore, some companies control employees' personal usage of the company's property including computer.

4. *"It's not easy to build windows using these new RAD tools."*
   This statement is true especially for GUI development tool vendors. If you know how to write short, effective code, it is sure productive to build windows using these new RAD tools.

5. *"The next version of the development tools will fix our current problems."*

It depends on what you have and how the vendor is going to upgrade it.

6. *"The manager does not need to know the methodology."*

   How can you supervise an accountant on the billing process if you do not know the billing process? If you are a manager, you need to know everything that will be required for a project.

7. *"We do not have to do any of this analysis and design stuff because we are going to purchase packages rather than build systems."*

   Coding may not need to be performed, however the system to by purchased must be analyzed to ensure the requirements of the business are met.

8. *"Standards will emerge as the project goes on."*

   The project may soon die if it starts with no standards. One can adapt standards established by another project and modify them for use on your project. Or, just create new standards for the project.

9. *"We need one standard methodology and one standard CASE tool."*

   A methodology includes group values, as well as roles, teams, activities, techniques, deliverables, and standards. It is a micro-culture embedded inside larger corporate and national cultures. If it does not fit the outer culture, it can be rejected. In the current client-server environment, hardware and software of different paradigms are used. One standard methodology is not always sufficient to solve a problem. Often more than one methodology is needed in order to complete a project. Some CASE tools have enough techniques and management tools built in to support a full life cycle methodology. It is important to keep in mind that methodology and CASE tools change over time.

RISKS OF CLIENT-SERVER DEVELOPMENT

Opportunities and risks are like two sides of a coin. The decision to adopt a client-server solution should be based on careful consideration of the following risks (Renaud, 1993; http://empire.lansing.cc.mi.us/course/wdavis/130/client_server.html; http://www. personal.kent.edu/~jnattey/spage7.html):

1. There is a common risk that technical management may overlook the capacity requirements of the system. This may cause unexpected failure in the future.

2. The client-server environment may be complex. The operation, maintenance, support, and administration of a large number of machines require consistent application of standard methods of implementation to keep the job manageable.

3. Some assumptions that were appropriate for a small network may not scale up well to a large network.

4. Poor deployment planning is a bad sign for managing client-server systems. Many IT managers are accustomed to only managing the host computer. This end-to-end system may be a challenge to IT management.

5. Management may face employees' resistance to the installation of new system and in coordination of installation activities.

6. Client-server system provides more flexibility on software applications for the requester/user. But, the user may frequently use two or three applications out of ten. The more flexibility the client-server system provides, the greater the chances for confusion by the user. Education on software applications may be required to train employees to effectively use the system.

7. Vendor competition can be a hidden and the biggest risk to business organizations utilizing client-server computing. Software Company A may buy out Software Company B & C to eliminate its competitors. Software Company A may stop supporting the X & Z applications sold by Software Company B & C later on for its own business purpose. The business organization buyers may have big problems when this situation happens.

FUTURE TRENDS IN CLIENT-SERVER COMPUTING

Information technology is a very volatile area that it is continuously and rapidly changing. Business strategies need to be changed as the information technology advances in order to make the business more competitive and keep up-to-date business information skills. The trend in the client-server environment can be looked at in two different ways. The "fat-client" approach is more favored in an environment where local access to the application is pertinent due its ability to provide user control over various software applications and its configuration.

On the other hand, thin client tends to be more favored by more structured business processes, where they prefer minimizing the costs on the fixed procedures and structures. A large healthcare organization is a good example of a business that may favor the thin client. Many healthcare organizations have fixed procedures and structured business environments. The implementation of thin client (fat server) may minimize their budget problems and provide better security and data controls regarding sensitive patent information. Since information sharing and building solutions are important functions of client-server computing and many businesses are expanding globally, it would not be surprising to see client-server computing, taking a step into the global business environment.

A HEALTHCARE INFORMATION SYSTEM APPLICATION

Healthcare information technology was an area that was a slow and quiet growing area a decade ago. There has been dramatic growth and internal expansion within information systems in healthcare since the Health Care Financing Administration (HCFA) established so many new rules and regulations to monitor and manage Medicare, Medicaid, and the whole healthcare system. Healthcare organizations need a system that can handle their growth easily and efficiently while meeting the stringent control and reporting requirements imposed by the government. Client-server computing can be an efficient tool for healthcare organizations' information systems needs.

One of the authors is working for a large county health and hospital system where a client-server architecture is gradually replacing the mainframe architecture. The current implementation includes a mainframe system called Patient Management/Patient Account System (PMAS) for all patient accounts, admissions, discharges, and transfers. The mainframe system (MDX) has been used by The Community Oriented Primary Care (COPC) to handle complete outpatient appointment, schedule, and account information for outpatient visits. MDX has been in use for about seven years and it currently does not have the capacity required for COPC to keep up with its patient information. MDX does not have the capacity for all outpatient information, so COPC can only keep its patient information for two years (from the current working day back to two years ago). Epic was selected to replace MDX. Epic is a client-server model and therefore, has client-server characteristics.

Like most other healthcare organizations, the one mentioned in this case study is not at the "bleeding-edge" of information technology. Over the intermediate term, this healthcare organization plans to utilize the PMAS system for all inpatient information and the Epic system for all outpatient use. Since the Epic system was recently installed and the client-server model has existed for several years, they are not likely to face a "technological crisis" until a new and improved efficient system is on the market.

SUMMARY AND CONCLUSION

Client-server computing offers businesses the potential for an increase in flexibility and cost effectiveness in processing, managing, storing and sharing data/information. But before a decision is made to implement client-server computing, many factors must be carefully considered. The technology continues to undergo rapid changes. For example, thin client-server computing is based on breakthrough technology that impacts the client, server and middleware components.

Therefore, it is essential in selecting a solution to a business' computing requirements that a system's approach is taken. First, the requirements must be established, not only current requirements, but forecasted long-term needs. Potential solutions, including client-server computing, need to be identified and evaluated with respect to performance, technology insertion, maintenance and support, training and total cost of ownership. This approach should reduce risks and provide management the ability for effective decision making over management issues that involve the distribution of data, data administration of data, location of processing functions, cross operating system integration, network capacity, and determining the software to be used to develop client-server applications.

REFERENCES

Haight, T. (1993). "The Steady Increase of Client/Server." *Client/server Computing:The Strategic Edge For A changing Landscape – A Supplement To Information Week*, vol.80.

Hachtel, G. (1994). "A Best of Breed Approach to Client/Server," *Data Management Review*, 4(1), 17-19.

Huff, Richard A. (1995). "Client/Server Technology: Is It A Bill of Goods?" *Information Strategy: The Executive's Journal*, 12(1), 21-28.

Diamond, Sidney (1995). "Client/Server: Myths & realities," *Journal of Systems Management*, 46(4), 44-48.

Parr, Harvey. (1995). "Can Client server live up to its promise?" *Insurance System Bulletin*, 11(4), 6-8.

Rifkin, Glenn (1994). "Information technology: The Client/server challenge," *Harvard Business Review*, v72n4, (Jul/Aug 1994), pp: 9-10.

Ramarapu, Narender K. "Client/server computing: Is it the right choice," *Information Strategy: The Executive's Journal*, 12(2), 39-41.

Renaud, Paul E. (1993). Introduction to Client/Server Systems. New York: John Wiley & Sons, Inc.

Ruble, David A. (1997). Practical Analysis & Design for Client/Server and GUI Systems. New Jersey: Prentice Hall, Inc.

Vaskevitch, David (1997). Client/Server Strategies. Boston Massachusetts: IDG Books Worldwide, Inc.

http://empire.lansing.cc.mi.us/course/wdavis/130/client_server.html

http://www.personal.kent.edu/~jnattey/spage7.html

About the Authors

Adi Armoni received his Ph.D. degree from the School of Business Administration at Tel-Aviv University in 1993. His dissertation deals with knowledge acquisition for Expert Systems. His bachelor degree is in Industrial Engineering, and his graduate degree is MBA with major in Information Systems, and Finance. Dr. Armoni serves as associate dean and head of the computer and information systems department at the College of Management, School of Business. His research interest focuses on strategic information systems, decision support systems, and healthcare information systems. He published many articles in major journals, serves as associate editor in four journals, and presents his research papers in international professional conferences.

Dr. Armoni is a senior consultant for companies all over the world, and specializes in strategic Information systems, information infrastructures and building effective executive information systems. Dr. Armoni also conducts projects for the World Bank in Eastern Europe and South America, in which he consults the local government in building information systems capacity, and developing the country's information infrastructure. Adi Armoni can be contacted by e-mail at <armonia@post.tau.ac.il>.

* * *

Sal Agnihothri is an Associate Professor of Operations Management in the School of Management at Binghamton University. Professor Agnihothri holds B.Sc. and M.Sc. degrees from Karnatak University, Dharwar, India, and M.S. and Ph.D. degrees from the University of Rochester. His current research interests are in the area of hospital operations, quality management, and field service operations. Professor Agnihothri has published in leading Operations Research and Operations Management journals such as *Operations Research, IIE Transactions, Naval Research Logistics, Computers and Operations Research,* and *Interfaces.* He is currently an Associate Editor of *Management Science.*

Ann Shou-an Char is a Systems Analyst at the Parkland Health & Hospital System in Dallas, Texas. She received a MBA in Health Services Management from the University of Dallas and is currently pursuing a second MBA in Information Technology on a part-time basis. She is a registered nurse in Taiwan and has worked for McKay Memorial Hospital in Taipei.

Aryya Gangopadhyay is an Assistant Professor of Information Systems at the University of Maryland Baltimore County (USA). His research interests include Electronic Commerce, multimedia databases, data warehousing and mining, and geographic information systems. He has authored and co-authored two books, numerous papers in journals such as *IEEE Computer, IEEE Transactions on Knowledge and Data Engineering, Journal of Management Information Systems,* and *ACM Journal on Multimedia Systems,* as well as presented papers in many national and international conferences. He can be reached at gangopad@umbc.edu.

Gehan Gunasekara teaches business law at The University of Auckland, New Zealand. He specializes in franchising, information and privacy laws. The particular focus of his research has been on the impact of new technology, including the impact of the Internet, on personal privacy. He is a contributor to several commercial law textbooks in New Zealand. His other areas of research include the techniques of judicial reasoning and media law. He has published articles in New Zealand and in the United Kingdom on the analogical use of statutes in developing the common law.

Richard Heeks (richard.heeks@man.ac.uk) is a Senior Lecturer in Information Systems at the University of Manchester, UK, in the Institute for Development Policy and Management: a postgraduate center for managers from developing and transitional economies. His most recently published book is *Reinventing Government in the Information Age* (Routledge, 1999). He has provided consultancy inputs to public sector and health organisations world-wide and currently directs a Masters program in Management and Information. His homepage is located at http://www.man.ac.uk/idpm.

Minh Q. Huynh earned his doctorate in Information Systems and his MBA at the School of Management, SUNY Binghamton. From Franklin and Marshall College he took a B.A. degree in Physics and from the University of Maryland a B.S. in Computer Science. Prior to his academic career, Minh had worked for the United States federal government for four years. His dissertation was concerned with "A Critical Study of Computer-Supported Collaborative Learning." His other research interests include application of social theory in IS research, the advancement of interpretive research, and healthcare information systems. So far he has published in the conference proceedings of the International Federation of Information Processing, International Resources Management Association, and North Eastern Decision Sciences Institute.

Lech J. Janczewski's (MEng, Warsaw; MASc, Toronto; DEng, Warsaw) over 30 years experience in information technology. He was the managing director of the largest IBM installation in Poland, and project manager of the first computing center in the Niger State of Nigeria. He is currently with the Department of Management Science and Information Systems of the University of Auckland, New Zealand. His area of research includes management of IS resources with the special emphasis on data security and information systems investments in underdeveloped countries. Dr. Janczewski has written more than 70 publications presented in scientific journals, conference proceedings and chapters in books. He is the chairperson of the New Zealand Information Security Forum and New Zealand Computer Society National Counsellor.

Anita Krabbel studied computer science at the universities Koblenz and Hamburg in Germany. From 1992 to 1997 she worked as a research assistant in the software technique group of the computer science department in Hamburg ,with the focus on evolutionary software development strategies and object-orientation for interactive application software. Besides working at the university, she was consulting for software companies in the domains hospital, local government administrations, banking and insurances. Since 1997 she has been a self-employed consultant. In her doctoral thesis she is working on domain analysis and modelling.

Bruno Lavi, B.A., MS.C., has 10 years experience in health systems, specializing in statistics and information systems. He received his MS.C. in Information Systems Management at the Leon Recanati Faculty of Management, Graduate School of Business & Administration at the Tel Aviv University, Israel. He earned his B.A. in Statistics at the Haifa University, Israel. Today he serves as the IS manager, specializing in Data Warehousing and Data Mining at the Sheba Medical Center in Israel. In addition, he is involved in several research studies regarding health and information systems. He also serves as an information systems consultant for various health organizations in Israel and abroad. Mr. Lavi is the co-author of several publications dealing with health system issues. He is considered a specialist in Data Warehousing and Data Mining projects for health systems in particular and he is often invited as a guest speaker in this field.

David Mundy (david.mundy@man.ac.uk) is a Lecturer in Information Systems at the University of Manchester, UK in the Institute for Development Policy and Management. He has considerable experience working with IT, and has conducted IT research and undertaken IT consultancy assignments in a number of countries.

Mahesh S. Raisinghani teaches Information Systems at the Graduate School of Management, University of Dallas. He is the chairman of the Electronic Commerce track a world representative for the International Resources Management Association, and has had numerous listings including the *Who's Who in Information Systems*, *Who's Who in the World* and *Who's Who Among Students in American Universities and Colleges*. Professor Raisinghani's previous publications have appeared in the *Journal of Information Systems Management, International Journal of Information Management, International Journal of Materials and Product Technology, Journal of Electronic Commerce, Journal of Information Technology Theory and Application, Industrial Management and Data Systems, Electronic Commerce World, Minority Business News USA*; chapters in *Annals of Cases in Information Technology Management and Managing Web-Enabled Technologies Application and Management: A Global Perspective*; and proceedings in several international, national and regional information systems conferences.

Zeev Rotstein, M.D., M.H.A., is currently Director of the Sheba Medical Center Acute Care Hospital in Israel. He received his M.D. from the Sackler School of Medicine at the Tel Aviv University and is board certified in Cardiology. He earned his Master's in Health System Management (M.H.A.) at the Leon Recanati Faculty of Management, Graduate School of Business Administration at the Tel Aviv University and is board certified in Health Care Administration. He is a Senior Lecturer the Sackler School of Medicine and the Leon Recanati Faculty of Management, Graduate School of Business & Administration, specializing in Health Systems Management. In addition he serves as a consultant to the Ministry of Health, Lombardia Region, Italy, and to the Ministry of Finance, Israel on health systems. He has been published dozens of times in medical and scientific journals, conference proceedings, collections of abstracts, written several chapters to books, and is the author of several papers invited at scientific meetings, as well as numerous other publications.

Angel Salazar (mbzajs@mail1.mcc.ac.uk) works from the UK as an international consultant in institutional development and health services management for developing countries. He has a Ph.D. in health informatics from Policy Research in Engineering, Science and Technology at the University of Manchester, UK. His professional and academic interests are health sector dynamics, innovations in health services management, management development and information systems strategies, and biomedical and clinical engineering.

Felix B. Tan is a Lecturer in Information Systems at The University of Auckland, New Zealand. He serves as the Editor-in-Chief of the *Journal of Global Information Management* and sits on the Editorial Board of the *Information Resources Management Journal*. His current research interests are in strategy-IT alignment, global information management and national information policy issues. He recently published a book, on IT Diffusion in the Asia Pacific. Prior to joining the university, he spent 10 years working in information systems management with an international shipping conglomerate and a multinational food manufacturing corporation, IT management consulting with Arthur Young, and was a Director of a private education center.

Ingrid Wetzel studied for the high school teaching profession in Mathematics, Protestant Theology and Music at the Johann Wolfgang Goethe-University, Frankfurt. After graduating in 1980 she worked in the computer department of a radio and television station in Hessen, studied Computer Science and worked as a research assistant in ESPRIT projects. After her diploma 1990, she was a member of the Database Group at Hamburg University. Since her doctoral degree in Computer Science in 1994, she is a member of the Software Engineering Group in Hamburg for a postdoctoral lecturing qualification. Her current research is in methods for CSCW, with a particular focus on participatory requirements engineering in organizations, cooperation modeling and design and implementation of group support technologies. Besides working at the university, she is consulting for software companies developing object-oriented software.

Index